CW01459978

The Wonder
and Happiness
of Being Old

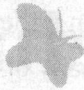

To my sister, Anne, the only person left who shares my memories (even if they differ), and to Mary, who lived so many of them with us, too.

The Wonder and Happiness of Being Old

Sophy
Burnham

BLUEBIRD

First published 2025 by Andrews McMeel Publishing

First published in the UK 2025 by Bluebird
an imprint of Pan Macmillan
The Smithson, 6 Briset Street, London EC1M 5NR
EU representative: Macmillan Publishers Ireland Ltd, 1st Floor,
The Liffey Trust Centre, 117–126 Sheriff Street Upper,
Dublin 1, D01 YC43
Associated companies throughout the world
www.panmacmillan.com

ISBN 978-1-0350-6285-0

Copyright © Sophy Burnham 2025

The right of Sophy Burnham to be identified as the
author of this work has been asserted by her in accordance
with the Copyright, Designs and Patents Act 1988.

All rights reserved. No part of this publication may be reproduced,
stored in a retrieval system, or transmitted, in any form, or by any means
(electronic, mechanical, photocopying, recording or otherwise)
without the prior written permission of the publisher.

Pan Macmillan does not have any control over, or any responsibility for,
any author or third-party websites referred to in or on this book.

1 3 5 7 9 8 6 4 2

A CIP catalogue record for this book is available from the British Library.

Printed and bound by CPI Group (UK) Ltd, Croydon, CR0 4YY

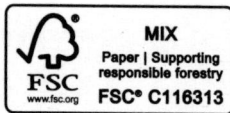

MIX
Paper | Supporting
responsible forestry
FSC
www.fsc.org
FSC® C116313

This book is sold subject to the condition that it shall not, by way of
trade or otherwise, be lent, hired out, or otherwise circulated without
the publisher's prior consent in any form of binding or cover other than
that in which it is published and without a similar condition including
this condition being imposed on the subsequent purchaser.

Visit **www.panmacmillan.com/bluebird** to read more about all our books
and to buy them. You will also find features, author interviews and
news of any author events, and you can sign up for e-newsletters
so that you're always first to hear about our new releases.

Tell all the truth but tell it slant—
Success in Circuit lies . . .

—*Emily Dickinson*

Contents

PROLOGUE

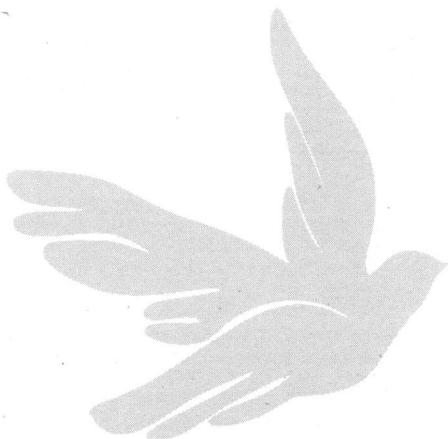

What's It Like to Be Old?

Dear Eleanor,

We were sitting in the sun at that lovely café on a side street in Paris, when you turned to me, appealing.

"I'm 59," you said with a haunted look. "In a few months I'll be 60." Then ducking your head shyly, "What's it like to be—"

You stopped. But I knew what you were too tactful to ask. What's it like to be *Old*?

"I'm afraid," you whispered.

Of course you are. Who wouldn't be afraid? You move now to the stage of "crone" and "hag." Fear is mostly what we hear about aging—fear of wrinkles; fear of loss; fear of diminishment; fear of humiliation and of being unwanted, abandoned; fear of the inexorable decline into chronic pain and death; fear of finding ourselves like King Lear, crying naked on the cliffs against the raging storm. It's fear exacerbated by a $48.4 billion beauty business pushing 18-year-old airbrushed skin as our ideal.

Who wouldn't be afraid?

I remember as I turned 60 asking my Aunt Kate that same question.

"What's it like in your 60s?"

She answered with a toss of her chin, visible even over the phone line: "Oh, Sophy, you won't even notice your 60s. Now at 90," she had murmured thoughtfully, "you begin to slow down."

She died at 103. That's forty more years along.

Sitting with you that day in Paris, I repeated her words. "Oh, Eleanor, you won't even notice your 60s. I bought my horse at 68. I stopped fox hunting at 80." (Mostly because of moving to Massachusetts, as it happens, but also because a fall when galloping to hounds is dangerous at my age—any age.)

The zeros are always scary. I remember being anxious when I reached 29 about turning 30—it felt so . . . old. I didn't celebrate my fiftieth birthday until, at 55, I threw myself a fiftieth, and then only for my closest friends. That's how ashamed I was of age. And afraid. Buried deep in our DNA is the memory of unwanted women burned at the stake as witches, or drowned (surviving proved them witches, to be killed again).

Sipping my espresso that warm September day, I thought how, at 85, this is one of the most interesting periods of my whole life. I have never felt so happy, so free. I wouldn't have missed it for the world. (Well, I would have, except my friend Death was elsewhere occupied.)

Now back home in Massachusetts, I keep musing on your question. What's it like to be old? At 85, I'm old. I'm told I'm old. I'm regarded as old. I don't feel old. I feel about 55.

So, I thought I'd try to answer your question.

Immediately, intellect rears up, scolding that mine is the experience of only one comfortably situated white woman living in America in this young century. How dare I say one word about aging? The subject is inchoate, chaotic, confusing. I am deeply aware of the sheer randomness of being born to the right circumstances. I could have been an impoverished woman in Mississippi, with the worst health care system in the world (equaled only by Mali in Africa!)— who could die from an abscessed tooth, if you can imagine, for lack of a dentist or of money to pay or transportation to reach one if she could. (So much is solved simply by money!) I could have been born a migrant fleeing torture or war or climate change, or else homeless, thrown begging on the streets by medical bills I could not pay. Twenty-five percent of seniors live on $15,000 or less, says Bernie Sanders. How dare I speak of the wonders of aging?

Sophy Burnham

But of course I will, because at my age, why not?

---

*A tale is but half told when
only one person tells it.*
—Saga of Grettir the Strong

When I was a little girl, I truly believed that 25 was old.
After that, nothing more happened in your life. You just went
on and on, trudging the same boring round of days with
nothing new to divert or delight. When I married at 23, my
5-year-old nephew turned my hand thoughtfully in his, as
if examining my lifeline, and murmured sadly, "When you
come back down the aisle, you'll be old."

I rather felt the same. After marriage I'd be a "matron."
And to show I'm not alone in this curious thinking, consider
one play by Beth Henley, in which the 30-year-old woman
is listed as a "matron." At 30! Oh, in my youth we had lots
of words to denigrate age: you were a spinster at 26. At 45,
unmarried, you were so old you'd become a failure. I
remember at 45 being surprised at how rich the world had
suddenly become.

So here I am, at 85, wading in the mud of old age. What do
I have to tell you, Eleanor, about being old?

It's not what you think. This is one of the happiest periods of my life. Perhaps the easiest way to tell you what it's like is to write about my days, recognizing that I am only one person, that each life is different, and each is fascinating right up to the end. Which may be another beginning, if what I hear is true, and noting also that even at this age, I still engage in denial, resentment, annoyance, indignation. I'm still learning—can you imagine? Wouldn't you think I'd have finished learning by now?

I may not send these letters to you. Perhaps they are principally for me, for I go along with E. M. Forster's statement: "How do I know what I think until I see what I say?"

Keep your heart high, Eleanor. It's not so bad.

Love,
Gophy

P.S. Here is a happy smile to lift your spirits: I found it in "Why Aging and Working Makes Us Happy in 4 Charts" in which researchers Carol Graham and Milena Nikolova find happiness increases with age. Note that the most difficult years come in your 40s and 50s.

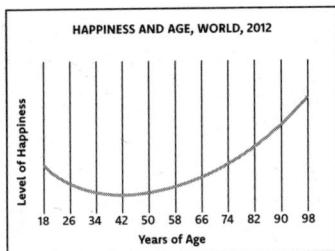

HAPPINESS AND AGE, WORLD, 2012

Level of Happiness

18 26 34 42 50 58 66 74 82 90 98
Years of Age

Apparently, happiness is not even dependent on finances and circumstances. It's an inside job. I remember my spiritual director once telling me about working in Bosnia during those terrible religious wars, where he was interviewing the homeless in tent-city concentration camps. He was awed by their courage.

"How can you be so happy?" he asked one toothless ancient crone who had lost everything. Sitting on the ground, she looked up at him, eyes sparkling. "Inside, I have hope."

P.S. Two thousand years ago, Cicero wrote a treatise on old age, *De Senectute*, which is well worth looking into now. "Enjoy the blessing of strength while you have it," he says, "and do not bewail it when it is gone, unless," he continues, "you believe that youth must lament the loss of infancy, or early manhood the passing of youth . . ." It's wry and witty, but I leave his delights to you.

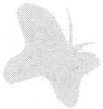

PART 1

I Hate Old Age

September 12

Dearest Eleanor,

Today I took a walk with my gang, all of them ten or twenty years younger than I. One woman brought along her mother, who at 89 is suffering with early dementia and who, unable to maintain her New York apartment or continue to teach at a university, has moved, unhappily, to her daughter's place up here in Massachusetts. It's hard for them both. The daughter gives up her privacy and social life to care for a mother made difficult by her fear and confusion, while the mother grieves for her independence and life in the city.

To my annoyance, I found myself walking with the mother for the full hour, simply because she stepped out as briskly as I, striding along, while the others strolled languidly behind, lost in conversation. I found myself irritated at being left to struggle with this old woman, whom I had never met before. I wanted the company of my younger friends, and there I was, stuck! We talked of her early life, which she could remember vividly, although a moment later she could not remember having just spoken of it. At the end of the walk,

I strode off, angry and upset with my gang, who had apparently grouped me with "aged." I don't want to be "old."

I despise "old"!

Age has no reality except in the physical world. The essence of a human being is resistant to the passage of time. Our inner lives are eternal, which is to say that our spirits remain as youthful and vigorous as when we were in full bloom.
Think of love as a state of grace, not the means to anything, but the alpha and omega. An end in itself.

—Gabriel García Márquez, *Love in the Time of Cholera*

As if to teach me a lesson, the Universe doubled down. After the walk came lunch with an acquaintance whom I'll call Cathy. It had been months since we two had seen one another, and I found myself once more shaken, impatient, and annoyed because Cathy can barely totter, even with the help of her cane. She is my age, our birthdays only days apart, but she has back problems, knee problems, balance problems, and especially problems with her negative outlook on the world. Clenching my teeth, I forced myself to slow down, take baby steps, hold Cathy's arm, open the door.

I watched the annoyance boiling in my breast, and at the same time I felt immensely grateful to be shown twice in the same morning the need for patience and also, more importantly, what awaits. Right now, I'm lucky that despite my chronological years, I'm not yet sick in body or mind.

Not yet.

But it will come, and like everyone in the world, I find myself sometimes straining for youth.

Remember the fairy tale about the old fisherman who captures a genie in a bottle? He's probably 45 or 50 in those long-ago times, but let's say he's 60. The genie gives him one wish. He thinks and thinks, standing on the seashore, examining his needs and what he wants: A new boat? Better fishing grounds? More money? And then, considering youth and his old, used-up wife, declares, "I'd like a wife thirty years younger than me."

"Done," says the genie. And poof! He's 90 years old.

Can you imagine how it would feel to wake up one morning and discover you were suddenly 80 or 85 or 90?

Fortunately, age sneaks up on little cat feet, and yet it always pounces by surprise.

Nothing is inherently and invincibly young except spirit.
And spirit can enter a human being perhaps better
in the quiet of old age and dwell there more
undisturbed than in the turmoil of adventure.

—George Santayana

As you see, Eleanor, I, too, am the product of my culture. I, too, am afraid of being "old." I pride myself that I'm not, but pride and arrogance cover denial and, of course, my own dislike, imbibed with conditioning. Meanwhile, I ride my horse. I work in my garden. I gather with loving daughters and with friends, and I still have strength and health and hair. And yet the numerals of my birth year shout to the world that I am "old." An elder, a crone, a Baba Yaga. The three sisters of Greek mythology, known as the Graeae, or gray-haired ones, were so old they could not remember such a thing as youth, so old they passed their one tooth and their one eye back and forth as needed. Two of their names were "alarm" and "dread."

That's what I think of when I think of "old."

Don't worry, Eleanor. You are only 60. You might live to 100. For that matter, given modern medicine, you could even live another 60 years. Some have. The famous French woman Jeanne Calment, born 1875, lived to 122 years and 164 days, dying in 1997. She is one of a few people verified to have lived to 120 and beyond. Another was the Muslim saint Hazrat Babajan, born at the turn of the nineteenth century, who died in 1931. Having achieved enlightenment in her 60s, she spent her years living on alms under a neem tree in India. There is also the Chinese Zen master Xuyun, or Empty Cloud, who lived for either 119 or 122 years. I remember reading about him in a book that unfortunately I've now lost. I was struck by the fact that he walked his whole life long, walking all around China and down into India and Southeast Asia, meditating and teaching. He never rode on a cart or horse but traveled only on his own two feet, unless crossing a river in a boat. Walking might be the fountain of youth. I don't know how much Jeanne Calment walked, but she never smoked, and she maintained a wide circle of friends.

My greatest beauty secret is being happy with myself.
—Tina Turner

The real question is what to do with this gift of time. In old age you know you are heading toward extinguishment. Each moment becomes precious, therefore, if only because of the darkening shadow at your shoulder. I am exquisitely aware that simply being alive is temporary—as is everything. Nothing is permanent, not even my beloved planet endlessly circling its star, which will itself implode, I'm told, in only another five billion years. Which may be why I'm so happy. I don't have time for the constant negativity and fear hammered and yammered at me by the media. That's for the young. They love to experience the adrenocortical jolt of fear.

Now I dash off to take care of the rest of the day, but always laughing at myself and life.

With love,
Sophy

Wisdom and Wonder

September 15

Good morning, Eleanor,

The thing that I notice most about getting old (and mind you, it is only this year that I begin to acknowledge "elder") is a loss of energy. Also of urgency. I don't move as quickly or gracefully as earlier. No one asks anymore if I used to be a dancer. It's not that I have lost curiosity or enthusiasm, but sometimes the expression of my happiness seems muted, like a faded color. The other day at the market I saw a young mother with two little girls of maybe 3 and 5. They were both hopping between the displays of vegetables, the piles of apples and pears, excited by the pyramids of oranges, hilltops of bottles, the wide, cold cases of cellophane-wrapped foods, everything coming as a surprise and object of delight. They would take a step and stop, almost overwhelmed by the riches spread before them, grab at each other's sleeve, "Look!"

And I thought, "Yes, that's what I've lost; it's that sense of wonder. It's the wild anticipation, when everything is new and possible and magical and never seen before."

By the time you get into your 80s, you have seen so much—no, I should say "I," speaking only for myself—that I find my mind comparing everything to something seen before, always comparing, judging, criticizing, analyzing, rather than simply attending with the attention of "shoshin," the quality that the Zen master Shunryu Suzuki calls "Beginner's Mind." With Beginner's Mind, you approach every situation with open-hearted eagerness and mindful lack of preconceptions, as if you have never seen it before. I notice now that even passersby on the street start to look like people I once knew, some of them long dead. I feel that nothing seems as fresh to me as to those bouncing little girls, and this is true despite the TV or papers shouting—no, screaming—about the latest catastrophic crisis. Creating anxiety and fear. I have learned that crises are nothing but challenges, and that Time has a way of working things out, if we just leave things alone. Even war has a way of working itself out, generally by exhaustion or attrition. One side wins and political conditions change, and power seeps like water in one direction or another. And then the cycle starts again.

> *O time, thou must untangle this, not I.*
> *It is too hard a knot for me t'untie.*
> —William Shakespeare, *Twelfth Night*

Is this inner stillness, this calming of energy, what they mean by wisdom? Yet I look at my two children and four grandchildren and feel they are all wiser than I have ever been. How do they know so much? Even my teenaged grandchildren are so open, searching, seeking, so involved and engaged in their experience! And moreover, so certain. I am deeply moved. I remember how once I, too, felt certain of everything. I had opinions!

Now I hardly understand anything at all.

You are not singular in suspecting
you know little. The longer I live,
the more I read, the more patiently
I think, and the more anxiously
I inquire; the less I seem to know.
—John Adams to his granddaughter
Caroline Amelia Smith de Windt, January 24, 1820

Having said I've lost the sense of urgent excitement, I'll add, Eleanor, that this loss—if it is loss—brings with it a great gift. These days I spend a lot of time just looking. I stand marveling at the purple tulip, that beautiful rock at the edge of the path, the blue jay at the bird bath—they take my breath away, not in the jumping-jack excitement of the two little girls at the market but with a deep stillness, like the

Sophy Burnham

profound black ocean waters that move far below the sparkling surface of bright waves.

It's not happiness.

I think it's joy.

As always,
Sophy

The Permanence of Love in a Temporary World

September 19

Dear Eleanor,

A few years ago, when I was 82, I fell madly, wildly in love with a man, a younger man—22 years younger to be exact—and I might mention it was also to my shame, because there is something unseemly about an old woman falling for a beautiful younger man, even if he is in his 60s. For more than two years we had the kind of restless love affair that made life as fascinating as if I were a teenager, and as uncertain. When you are in love, everything feels new and beautiful. You rise up on emotional tiptoe, and it doesn't matter whether you are 18 or 80. I woke up each day in anticipation of what might happen next. I felt alive.

Aging and sex. That's a big topic. I may talk more about that later. Or not. As for my love affair, we broke up after two years, right on schedule. I spent most of the next year grieving, and now I'm OK again, but I sometimes feel the letdown, an absence of that flood of dopamine and norepinephrine in my brain. Maybe what I'm saying is only that I feel restless these days or mildly discontent. Yet I had that love, and thinking of him makes me happy, without needing to reach out to him again. Mostly, I am glad to be alive and also, I might add, without pain (minor aches don't count), but neither am I wildly in love, and I miss that giddy, heightened joy.

Does that have anything to do with age? Doesn't everyone feel a letdown when a love breaks up? Or at the loss of one you loved?

Recently, we met by accident on the street, and I felt my heart rise up toward him with happiness, my eyes taking pleasure in his beauty and grace. Our eyes met. In that moment I knew he loves me still. No question that I am loved. We spoke a few words, touched fingers, parted, and for a full day I have found myself daydreaming and longing. Could we get back together? Would it "work" this time? Love demands union, communion. But the longing means only that I love, in the same way that when I miss my grandchildren (who have their own rich teenage lives and give no thought to an old granny), it means only that I love. And yes, I choose the loss that means I love.

Loss colors all our lives. As soon as we discover something of value, we're afraid of losing it. Yet life is nothing but loss, beginning with the loss of safe, warm darkness at birth, when comfort explodes in light and noise, the loss of childhood, loss of innocence, loss of friends and much-loved animals, the loss of brothers, mother, father, loss of investments, the loss of homes with their creaking floorboards and cribs and cozy nooks, loss of jobs and marriages, loss of children, loss of dreams, and the repeated loss of self-esteem, and always hanging over us the loss of self that will be produced by death. Which is to say the extinction (for us) of the entire world.

Nothing is sweeter than love, nothing higher, nothing stronger, nothing larger, nothing more joyful, nothing fuller, and nothing better in heaven or on earth.

—Thomas à Kempis, fifteenth-century scholar, *The Imitation of Christ*

It isn't loss that's bad. It's how we deal with it. That's what I mean, Eleanor, about knowing that everything is temporary. Even this body that I inhabit. It's rented. I live in it like a suitcase, which gets so beat up over the decades that eventually it's uninhabitable; and then I'll pull myself out, like a white shirt waving in the breeze, and I'll move on. I'm told I can always rent another, if I like.

Being and Doing

Dear Eleanor,

Once I met the 96-year-old grandmother of a Virginia friend. She was working in her hot garden at the time, wearing a shapeless cotton dress and a wide-brimmed hat. She put down her shovel with a welcoming smile, dusted her hands on her dress, and invited us inside for cookies and lemonade. She announced that she'd just converted to Christian Science. "It's all about mind over matter," she said. "What you think is what you get."

At the time I chuckled in sarcastic derision. I hadn't yet read the *Bhagavad Gita* or the Buddha's *Dhammapada*. Much less the New Thought spiritual movement of the American 1880s. I knew nothing about the power of the mind or about intention and thought. I knew nothing yet of healing energy. Today, I have my own way of expressing it: so generous is the Universe, I now believe, so loving are the angels that surround us, that they bring all the desires of our hearts; happiness to those who think kind, generous, optimistic thoughts; sorrow to those who prefer fear, anger, hopelessness, victimization, and pain.

What you think is what you get.

Of course it's not as simple as that. Let's talk about that when I see you next.

We are what we think
All that we are arises with our thought.
With our thoughts we make the world.
Think and act with an impure mind and trouble
*   will follow you*
As the wheel follows the ox that draws the cart.

We are what we think
All that we are arises with our thought
With our thoughts we make the world.
Speak or act with a pure mind
And happiness will follow you
As your shadow, unshakable.

—The Dhammapada

My children tell me I'm always moving, active, that I never sit down. But often these days, I am content just to lie on the couch, reading. Or playing chess puzzles on the internet, trying to improve my game.

Being at this age takes up a good deal of my time, by which I mean just listening, looking—as if I must soak each moment in, memorize this world before I leave.

Here's another thing that's different from when I was young.

Deep inside, consumed, I suppose, at the table of family and culture, I learned that Doing or Creating has more value than indolent Being. Life itself reinforces the lesson, when holding down a job, caring for kids and dogs and house and partner and often for ailing parents at the same time, leaves no room even to take a bath without interruption, much less a whistle-blown time out. Sometimes, even at 85, I feel the familiar quickening of guilt that I should be putting even Looking to good use. I should paint or write or sew, or strive to leave some immortal work, and supposedly that would be "better."

Today I find that I don't care to hold onto the moment. Not only is it impossible but even morally wrong to try to dam the rushing river of time. Nor do I long to represent the world anymore in paint or unpublished words—trash for others to toss out when I leave.

Letters are signs of things, symbols of words, whose power is so great that without a voice they speak to us the words of the absent, for they introduce words by the eye, not by the ear.

—Isidore of Seville, seventh-century scholar, *Etyumologiae*, Book I, ch 3

This marks a huge difference from earlier in my life, when I strove to leave a trace of having lived. (In my dream it was a book that someone fifty or a hundred years after my death would read and pass on with delight to their children's children, before it crumbled into dust. I wanted that teensy immortality.)

Now, to live unknown, unnoticed, seems luxurious—like dying—anonymously and quietly recycling this body back to tender earth. That's how most people have died, after all, since long before the earliest Ice Ages four hundred thousand years ago, each beloved individual leaving no trace behind.

Today the idea seems correct and right and even beautiful.

The word "school" is taken from the old Greek *schole*, meaning "leisure." Aristotle saw contemplation as the highest human activity and thus essential to happiness. "For we do business," he said, "in order that we may have leisure." The point of leisure is to become more fully human. It is not the same as indolence, or even rest. It may even entail some "work." Leisure offers space to discover who we are and who we want to be, where we stand in the world, and what things we value.

What I'm trying to say, Eleanor, is that old age is not a punishment, and neither is it the end of new stories. Rather, with leisure, which is to say with Being, it points toward a new flourishing and flowering, like the trees in autumn that turn a ferocious blaze of colors, overwhelming us with beauty before they drop their leaves.

When I was young, I was driven to write. Indeed, I remember clearly the single moment I chose to be a writer, an artist, a storyteller. I was probably 12, curled up in my father's big chair in the study and reading the *Iliad*. Homer was describing the death of one hero when he wrote that to die in battle is the finest death a man can achieve, his name ringing down the corridors of time, immortal.

I dropped the book, appalled.

That's not what I want, I thought. I want to be the one who writes about it in such a way that three thousand years later a little child (me) deciphering black worm-squiggles on a white page is moved to tears or laughter by the singer now long dead. That's what I want! Nothing less than immortality. And I wanted it so much that I couldn't tell anyone, except God, perhaps, in my secret prayers. What I wanted in my writing was, in the words of Tacitus, "to touch the minds and hearts of people everywhere." At the same time, I didn't dare to put pencil to paper until well into my 20s: it was too BIG. How could I compete against Dostoevsky or Tolstoy or Jane Austen or George Eliot or the so-many-others who captivated me? (I never considered that most were writing only seventy or eighty years earlier. Or that they struggled. Or rewrote.)

I've been lucky. I have enjoyed success; my books and talks have affected people all over the world. I have even had my fifteen minutes of celebrity (horrible!), as Andy Warhol playfully suggests everyone gets.

At one time I was so driven that it was one of the several forces breaking up my family. I chose to write.

Now quietude, just Being, seems enough.

Is that the wisdom of age? Or is it simply that I don't have the energy anymore for all that flurry?

Our best activity is the contemplation of the wonders of things and it takes huge qualities of soul, intellect, and character to spend much time wondering and contemplating the beauty.

—Aristotle, *Nicomachean Ethics*

For the first time in my life, I'm not driven. Neither do I feel the need for outside acknowledgment. What I want now, at this tender elder-age, is simply TO BE.

That's one big change, Eleanor, that has come in my 80s. I'm sure there are more.

And yet Being, too, requires practice. I was talking with a friend last night—and another lovely thing about this time of my life, Eleanor, is that conversations so often run into deep channels, often unexplored, as if we don't have time anymore for superficialities. It is curious how quickly we move straight to what is bothering us.

> *Beautiful young people*
> *are accidents of nature, but beautiful*
> *old people are works of art.*
> —Eleanor Roosevelt

"I find this a confusing time," she said. "Who am I now? What am I here for? I'm not working anymore. My life has shrunk; it's smaller," she said gesturing with both hands as if to enclose herself in narrowing walls. "But I see more clearly, and friendships—even in my exercise class I'm meeting these other women, and they are so interesting! I met a woman who got her grad degree, not even a PhD, and was working on AI in the 1970s! I didn't take time before—it would not have occurred to me to learn about other people. I mean, I socialized but usually for work, and it was all about efficiency, and always with some goal in mind."

22

And then we got down into the nitty-gritty about Doing and Being, because she is a working artist, while the third in our coven of witches who meet each week is a playwright and opera librettist, and so we are all Doing and creating, in spite of thinking that in these years we spend all our time just Being.

All my love,
Sophy

Oh, the Little Humiliations

Dearest Eleanor,

The knees are the first to go, but that can happen in your 40s or 50s—or earlier, if you've had an accident. If it's not the knees, it's the hips or else the back. My osteopath says that humans stood up ten thousand years too soon. Even a dog or a horse gets arthritis, and to have it in my back and hip does not seem surprising after years of running, skipping, skiing, riding, twirling, playing, dancing, working, constructing, laboring. What beautiful bodies we live inside of! What amazing, self-healing organisms! A heart, that secret turbine, beats 60 or 70 times a minute: 86,400 times a day, 31,536,000 times a year without a pause; and it does this year after year after year, never stopping, never gasping. In eighty-five years, mine has beaten 2.5704 times carried to the ninth power. And I don't have to do anything, Eleanor, can you believe it?—not count, not concentrate, not climb sleepily out of bed at two in the morning to click a switch or push a button. I do nothing. Like-wise, the lungs draw in air and let it out every few seconds, each breath coursing oxygen through the brilliant blood of my body.

And they say there are no miracles! Each breath is different, long, short, slow, fast, hurried or quiet, elegant or ragged. I think if we deeply listened to our bodies, we would be so overcome with gratitude—and love—and love for the magnificent instrument we live inside of that has served us so long and well—that we couldn't ever be afraid of age.

Our concept of "aging" is governed more by fear than by the passage of years. I know people who play tennis in their 90s or picked up golf in their 80s. I was reading the other day about the neurologist and Nobel prize laureate Rita Levi-Montalcini, who discovered that neurons in the brain regenerate and regrow. New hands or arms or legs can't regrow, in the way of an octopus's limb, but the nerves in our brains replace themselves. Think of that. They need to be exercised, of course. Levi-Montalcini worked right up to the age of 100. She died in 2012 at age 103. Concerning mental exercising, by the way, there's the story of the former law clerk who went to visit his old friend Supreme Court Justice Oliver Wendell Holmes Jr., then in his 90s. He found the venerable old man surrounded by papers on the floor.

"What in the world are you doing?"

"I'm learning Greek," Holmes answered. "The mind is just another muscle. You have to exercise the mind."

At one point, when in his 60s, Joseph Fuchs, the violinist, who is known for his vigorous playing with rich, warm tones, lost the use of the fingers in his left hand. He could no longer play. He taught himself to use his fingers in a new way, and in his 90s gave a one-man concert at Carnegie Hall.

But I was talking of the little humiliations. My ribs sit on my hip bones at this age, so much have I shrunk; my breasts sink to what used to be my waist. My skin has become tissue-paper thin, raising purple bruises on my forearms just by the weight of my purse. God help me if I bump a doorjamb. My bladder leaks. I need to wear a pad. I have to pee so often that I find myself keeping one eye peeled for restroom. Everyone has twinges. Aches. Your ankle hurts. Or your shoulder. Or hip. Or back. At night you wake up gasping from the cramp in your foot and have to get out of bed to walk around for a minute. (Magnesium helps, I'm told. Or eat two Brazil nuts a day.)

Maybe this—and pain—is what we're thinking of when we think of age. Yet pain can attack at any age, the result of accidents or wars.

I know a woman who at the age of 17 was paralyzed in a car crash from the armpits down. She went on to graduate from college, then graduate school, went on to law school, and finally to become a federal judge. She travels. She skis. She is bold and brilliant, but remember, though in a wheelchair, she's not in pain. (Except lifting and lugging the wheelchair around: that's hard.)

Pain hits every age.

> *. . . it happens fast for some people and slow for some, accidents or gravity, but we all end up mutilated. Most women know this feeling of being more and more invisible every day.*
>
> —Chuck Palahniuk, *Invisible Monsters*

Moving helps. We are animals. We are born to keep moving. My doctor says that moving scrapes away the rust. Walking. Dancing. Doing yoga, energy work, Tai Chi, qigong, riding my horse, working in the garden. Just keep moving, Eleanor, while you can. Without abusing yourself. This, and a good diet, staves off the worst, though in the end of course no one gets out of life alive. I won't say anything about addictions. Obviously, drugs will drag you down.

Emotional pain is equally degrading. The loss of your wife or husband of sixty years can make you old in a minute.

It's not only in your head. Heartbroken, you wake up old.

Mirrors

September 28

Dear Eleanor,

Today I had a hot rock Ayurvedic massage, and it left me limp on the heated table, my mind moving idly in a kind of hypnogogic haze until my face, as seen this morning in a public restroom mirror, jolted me. The lighting was cruel, and every wrinkle, fold, and sag showed with alarming clarity. The lighting in my home bathroom is more tender. It shields me from what others probably note every day. Moreover, my eyes, which peer outward from behind my face, encourage the deceit that I am still young, without wrinkles—which, after all, was the reality for most of my life. It is certainly the reality inside. Inside, I'm only 40 or 50.

The tragedy of old age is not that one is old,
but that one is young.

—Oscar Wilde, *The Picture of Dorian Gray*

One day my granddaughter, then 16, confessed that she hated herself when she looked in the mirror, but if she imagined she were looking at someone else, either a stranger or a friend, she found the image very pretty.

There's a lesson in that.

People compliment me on how well I look, and some give a great beaming smile on hearing my age: "NO! I don't believe it! You look twenty years younger!" I happily accept the flattery, and in my mind's eye I don't think they're wrong. Which made it all the more startling this morning to view myself in the harsh light of that restaurant restroom. Myself, now "Old."

When I was little, we had roughly three mirrors in the whole house. If I wanted to see what I looked like, I had to climb up onto the bathroom sink to look into the medicine cabinet mirror set high on the wall.

The lack of mirrors may have been deliberate. Vanity was not encouraged in my family. My sister and I were never told that we were pretty—nor, for that matter, not. Beauty was far down on the scale of accomplishments. Nonetheless by the time I was 5, it had somehow come to my notice that beauty equals love. Could I be loved?

It's a strange question, when I knew I was loved. I was the middle child and, therefore, competing against two others for our mother's time and attention. As the second child, I was supposed to have been a boy, a disappointment right from birth. Yet we children were loved, two girls and our little brother, who came along later, the prince. In my family, we never hugged or kissed or even touched (as happens now even with minor acquaintances); we never said "I love you" to each another. Yet I never doubted I was loved. Indeed, I felt the trees above me bend down as I played under them, watching tenderly, loving me. As a child, I felt the air filled with light and wild colors and the silent song of angels, and I still remember my heart opening one day, arms flung wide, pouring my love out onto the light-struck grass and moss and trees and even onto the corner of the brick house, all of them loving me back.

Yet somehow, contradictory as it sounds, I also understood that I had to earn approval. Somehow, without anyone telling me, and despite my mother's best efforts at hiding the mirrors, by age 5 I knew that "pretty" won.

This is just to say that I have always been vain, which is why I find it difficult today to see my wrinkles and sagging breasts and bulging belly. I fight against aging. I watch myself resist, deny my years, and take pride in being called twenty years younger.

The Buddha notes that pain and suffering are different. You can have pain, but you don't need to wallow in it and thereby create suffering. I guess in reaching these years I finally start to learn the meaning of letting go, let go and let God, to observe without demanding anything.

Suffering lies in resistance, either by disliking what you have or desiring what you don't think you have.

So in this period of aging, I get once more to observe this continual egotistic shifting between desire and dislike. I get to watch my vanity, this time with amused recognition and even loving generosity. I also get, rebelling, to throw away makeup and hair coloring and creams and all the products I used to spend so much money on in order to be admired or to attract a man; these days I get to toss out even the care I once lavished on clothes, since everyone in my town wears jeans and the weather, moreover, is so cold in winter (and spring and fall) as to require layers of down. We all look like the Michelin Man. It's another liberation.

The great secret that all old people share is that you really haven't changed in seventy or eighty years. Your body changes, but you don't change at all. And that, of course, causes great confusion.
—Doris Lessing

If you didn't know I was a woman, would you think me a man? Our bodies bulk out as we age, pear shaped. Everything droops. We pluck hairs from our chin at the same time that hairs vanish at the armpits or crotch. We become like children again, and sometimes (when I'm in a ready mood) I feel myself about 9 years old, throwing my love extravagantly, arms flung wide, onto the tender ginger cat, the grass, the squirrel spiraling up the tree, tail quivering, the autumn ginkgo, so butter yellow I can taste the color, the woods, the rocks, and love pouring out onto that woman grappling with her shopping cart as she grabs her screaming child, shushing him in her shamed desire to present a public face.

How beautiful is this prideful struggle that means we're still alive.

Meanwhile, it's a good idea to put the mirrors too high on the wall to look into. That way, I'm always "me."

Taking the Dare

October 4

Dear Eleanor,

Last December, when I turned 85, I promised myself I wouldn't take my horse over jumps anymore. A rather serious fall earlier that year had brought to my notice that, at my age, a fall from horseback invites a broken hip or neck or death or, even worse, paralysis. But a week ago, riding out alone, I couldn't resist the temptation of taking a tiny crossbar, and I could feel my horse's delight, her ears pricked in attention as I guided her toward the jump. She sailed over it, galloping afterward with sheer joy, and the next day I asked Kate to give me a jumping lesson over the full course of jumps.

Why a lesson?

Because I don't want to jump alone. Because even after years of riding, I feel safer and braver with an instructor.

I haven't told you about my beautiful Arab mare, Spring. I bought her in New Mexico when I was 68 and she was only 4. (There's optimism for you.) It was not that I was looking for a horse. In fact, what I'd been praying for was a man, someone to share my life. God works in mysterious ways. Then I met Spring, a pretty black 3-year-old with one white hoof and a star on her forehead. She was the most intelligent, willing, forward, courageous horse I'd ever met, and she trusted me completely. Still, I didn't want a horse. Horses are expensive. I divided my time between New Mexico and Washington, D.C. Someone else bought her, and that summer when she was 3, I leased and rode her whenever I was in New Mexico. A perfect solution.

Then something happened. Back in Washington, I woke up one December morning with a clear "Knowing" that Spring, out in New Mexico, would be sold and moved to Portland. I would never see her again.

I called the stable.

"If Spring is ever for sale," I said after initial courtesies, "do let me know."

"Strange that you should say that. Her owner called me only yesterday to say she has to move to Portland, Oregon, and needs to sell Spring."

For months I bargained with God. I didn't want a horse. A horse is expensive. How would I ever afford a horse? Moreover, she would always be across the country, wherever I wasn't. . . . Finally, I remembered the adage "All things are possible with God." If the Universe, God, my guardian spirits, wanted me to own Spring, it would bring me the money to afford her. Somehow, against all evidence, I am supposed to TRUST.

The decision was made easier by remembering one earlier time when I had felt similarly directed to do something that Reason opposed. At that time, I had been praying for direction in a period when I felt particularly lost, unglued. "God, help me. Show me what I'm to do next, how to be of service. Help." Again, I had woken up again with the clarity of a "Knowing," as if I'd heard a voice: New York City, six months, followed by a joyful "YES!"

This joy, this "Yes" is always one of my signs of God.

Of course, I instantly gave in to doubt. "New York City! I can't afford New York. Why go there?" Etc. etc., ad nauseum, until once more I reminded myself: "All things are possible with God."

That day I telephoned three people I knew in New York, asking if anyone knew of a sublet for four or five months (already bargaining, you see). One directed me to her friend Charlotte. I left a message for Charlotte on her office voice-mail. That morning as Charlotte picked up her mail in her building at 66th and 2nd Avenue, a woman approached.

"You're a real estate agent?" she asked. "My friend Mary just died, and the family want to rent her two-bedroom, rent-controlled, furnished apartment for six months. Would you know of someone?" When Charlotte reached her office, there was my call, asking for just that.

I questioned daily why I came to New York, but I became friends with Charlotte, who, it turned out, was dying. We spent hours talking about death and illness and life. It was also in those months that I learned I was a medium and psychic.

So, remembering to trust the Universe, I bought Spring. We have ridden across the New Mexico mesa and high into the fragrant, pine-scented mountains, we have foxhunted in Virginia (she loved it), and we've won ribbons in horse shows or doing dressage. She is the love of my heart, and she loves me in return.

So today I took Spring over the jumps at the stable here in Massachusetts.

It was a glorious blue-sky Indian-summer day. I had already walked and trotted her over poles laid on the ground to warm her up, loosen her joints. Then we took almost every jump in the field, and I felt triumphant! And so did she. Spring loves to jump, and she loves to work out the intellectual puzzle of cantering from one jump to the next, judging distance and height and getting the footing right. Kate, the stable owner, texted me later, "You're fabulous!" I preened under the praise, ignoring the implication that the fabulosity refers to jumping at my age. Back to Aging, you see. At 85, I'm not supposed to jump. Or maybe she said it because I am one of the few at the stable who dares to jump. The others ride walk-trot-canter round the arenas. Most are afraid even to hack out, riding in the beautiful woods with other horses, much less alone.

Afterward my knees ached from the unaccustomed exercise. I may never jump again. I probably won't, because already I feel my body refusing to be able to do the things I like. Still, I never want to reach my deathbed and think, "I could have done it, and I didn't take the dare." Better to try and fail. And fail again. And fail another time, rather than to give up without even trying, especially by using the age card, "I'm too old."

What I'm saying, Eleanor, is say yes to life. Gobble it up while you can. You get so much by simply being brave.

. . . be on the alert to recognize your prime
at whatever time of your life it may occur.

—Muriel Spark

Family Anger

Dearest Eleanor,

I'm sitting outside on the deck on this sunny day. The leaves are falling, red and golden brown. Down the cliff someone at the high school is practicing on drums for band, and it's pleasant to sit here in the warm light before the time when the sun goes behind the roof and I am driven back indoors by cold.

What I notice about aging is how gradually, almost without thinking about it, things drift away. I don't go out dancing anymore. I don't do yoga as religiously as I used to, or ski, or skate. I still work in the garden. I heave boxes around and clean the garage, or oil the new deck, or clean the basement, or muck out the horse's stall. It's the things I don't do that go unnoticed. The last time I took out my bike, I turned the wheel too quickly, fell, and scraped my knee and hands, gravel embedded in my palm. It's not that I made a decision not to bike, but rather it has lost its flavor.

While speaking of flavor, I should note that I have lost my sense of smell. I can't smell the lilies of the valley at my doorstep, or the lilacs. Friends say, "Oh, smell the honey-suckle." But I can't. It's like my hearing. Even with hearing aids, I no longer hear birdsong. And that's a sorrow. Then let's not forget the tongue. Oh dear, the tongue. How loose it gets with age.

We all hear about the lack of inhibition that comes with age. It's a cultural joke—the aging grandmother who blurts out the forbidden truth or starts swearing when she never cursed in her life. I have spent a lifetime trying to learn how to speak (or, God help me, not to). By nature, I am tactless, forthright. It has taken years to understand that other people don't always want to hear the truth, my truth. Moreover, in my family—yours, too, Eleanor—most ordinary conversation might best be named "Blurt." Like your grandmother, my Aunt Eleanor, who, on seeing my teenage daughter Molly with a nose ring, snuffled, "Oink-oink."

Forty years later, the insult still scalds Molly. She mentioned it just the other day.

At the age of 40 I started to teach myself to speak. I wanted to express myself with such care that the other person could actually hear what I wanted to say. This meant being aware of the other person and adjusting my voice and body language. It meant choosing different words for different persons and even different tones of voice. Now, forty years further on this journey, I sometimes find myself impatient, as if I don't have time anymore for courtesies. Screw them. Let them accommodate to me! Let me shine forth, with all my flaws and failings, and let the pieces fall where they may.

Here's an example. I mentioned walking once a week with the small group of friends. One I will call Caroline, who is so private and reserved that she barely speaks. A few months ago, I found myself hiking with her far ahead of the others, and wishing to know her better, I revealed a confidence in hopes it might encourage a deeper intimacy. She shrugged, unresponsive, hiking on. She said nothing. I couldn't believe it. I felt my gorge rising. I stopped and lit into her, raging, about how much her insensitivity hurt.

"Well . . .," she said. And set off up the hillside as fast as her long legs could take her, and since then, we have stepped around each other like enemy dogs, careful never to be alone without the protection of the group.

I don't like her.

The point is that not so long ago I would probably not have reached out to her in the first place, but neither would I have revealed my hurt. Much less my anger.

If the heart of one friend is open to another, the
truth glows between them, the good enfolds them,
and each becomes a mainstay to his companions,
a helpmate . . . . There is nothing surprising in this:
souls ignite one another, minds fertilize one another,
tongues exchange confidences; and the mysteries
of this human being . . . abound and spread.

—Abu Sulayman al-Sijistani, tenth-century Islamic philosopher

Writing this, recognizing my hurt and anger, I realize (oh, darn it!) now I have to pray for her for two weeks (yes, fourteen days), offering in my imagination everything that I, myself, have ever wanted and everything that I think she might want. I need, as Christ says, to forgive her. I need to slither out of my selfish annoyance and self-pity and recognize that she, like every one of us, is also hurting. Trying to survive.

The prayer is not for her, of course. It's for me. It's to release myself from the prison of disgruntlement and dislike. And I don't need to spend much time doing it—a thought flung out, a moment of generous good will: that's enough. But I must do it every day. It takes two weeks sometimes. And in my hurt or anger, if I can't bring myself to the depths of heartfelt prayer, then just begin: "God, help me to forgive." Implicit is my other desire: "God, help me to forgive myself. Help me to love again."

You grew up in this same culture, Eleanor, so you'll remember how important it was in our family to be proper, how important especially for your grandmother, my Aunt Eleanor, who was married to the Admiral, to present a brave and seemly face to the world. Never show yourself vulnerable. Never out of control. And never, under any circumstances, show anger or rudeness in public! I wrote in my book *The Landed Gentry* a little about this WASP discipline. Maybe, being the younger generation, you'd already tossed out this Edwardian reserve, but it was strict for us children, my siblings, my cousins, and me.

It never occurred to me when I was a child that the adults, laughing like booming giants high over my head, ever felt fear or jealousy or hurt or anger or anxiety. Oh, how they laughed and played—how they played! Riotously enjoying one another. Meanwhile, we children had rules. And often we learned them by osmosis. By making a mistake. Once learned, the next reproof might be no more than one raised finger or the Look to make us fall into line. We learned early never to interrupt or insert a question or comment into adult talk.

It's curious how, looking back over my life, I see, like watching a movie, the long-dead older generation move through their houses. I can almost hear their footsteps, nearly make out what they are calling about. Everything happens in memory all at once, time having no chronological order, so that one moment I'm 10 years old, reading *Ferdinand the Bull* in Aunt Kate's two-room apartment over the garage at Gaga's farm, and the next I'm 15, filling my fine Spode china plate with tuna casserole from Aunt Eleanor's Hepplewhite sideboard and carefully carrying it to the lace place mats waiting with the heavy silverware on the mahogany table for lunch.

It's curious how I remember them in the prime of their lives, not when I've grown to adulthood and become their equals, as it were, and not when they, at the end, have diminished into the tragedy of old age. In my memory, they are always young.

Back to Anger.

I'm told that when I was very little, perhaps 1 or 2 years old, I would get so angry I'd hold my breath. (Did I scream as well? It's not part of the family story.) What my mother did (frightened, alone, with two children) was grab a glass of water and throw it in my face. I would gasp, gulp, breathe in . . . and everything would return to quiet again. I'm told my mother had only to take one step toward the kitchen sink and I would choke back to propriety. I don't remember this, but she was proud enough of her solution to make it a family story.

I've often wondered, especially once I had my own children, why she didn't take me into her arms, hug, or comfort me? What I learned, though, from that early age is that, while others could, I was not allowed To Be Angry. All my life, I have tried to stifle anger. (David, my ex, would dispute this, but that's another story.) I will leave a room to calm down, or take a walk, or hang up on you on the phone—anything rather than explode with the dangerous sensations rising in my breast.

One day—and I was in my 50s at the time—I was eating lunch with a good friend at a restaurant in Santa Fe (imagine the quiet clink of cutlery, the white tablecloths, the waiters soundlessly filling water glasses). We were both furious. It had been a hard afternoon together, and she was as upset with me as I with her. I remember seething in stifled silence as she pecked at me. Until I grew so angry that suddenly I picked up the glass of water at my place mat—and threw it in my face!

"Oh, you're so dramatic," she said.

But I was hit by illumination. In that moment everything fell into place: my mother's fearful water-dousing when I was little, my inability all my life to admit anger (I called it annoyance, irritation), much less express it openly. After that I have been able to release my anger—as with poor Caroline on that walk—though I still try to keep it on a leash.

Ah well, perhaps one has to be very old before one learns how to be amused rather than shocked.

—Pearl S. Buck, *China Past and Present*

My friend Sherry married five times (but twice to the same man, so she counted them as only four). One day she grew so angry at her latest husband that, remembering her therapist's injunction to express her anger, she threw all his belongings out on the street: clothes, furniture, books, papers, typewriter, shoes, underwear, coffeepot, everything of his.

To her surprise, when he came home, he simply hauled it away.

The next day she came over to sit in my garden with me, our iced tea glasses sweating in the summer heat.

"I don't think she should have told me that, do you?" Sherry complained. "I didn't mean for him to leave."

I guess it wasn't the worst thing to be taught the dangers of unleashed anger. We argued in our family, discussed and disputed in intellectual battles. But rarely were emotions mentioned. One day I came down to the breakfast table, where Daddy sat at his end of the table, reading the paper, while Mummy, at the opposite end, had a quiet moment to herself. I remember murmuring, "I don't feel well."

"Well, don't tell anyone," my mother snapped. "No one wants to hear."

My father looked up, surprised. "That's not true," he said. But it was my mother's voice I heard.

Today, looking back from seven more decades of experience, my heart goes out to my mother; for all her life she suffered from eczema so serious that as a child she had scratched away the entire outer epidermis, the skin on her arms and chest and face. This was before penicillin, cortisones, and modern medications. She had learned from earliest childhood to endure, that no one could do anything about her pain, that no one wanted to hear. Looking back, I think she was one of the bravest people I have ever met.

The Beauty of Age

Dear Eleanor,

I have just been given the most astonishing birthday present! I can't believe it. I keep going over the events, as if to find a crack in the cement, something to mar this beautiful and encouraging moment. I've told you how I feel, Eleanor, in my deepest heart about old age—how ashamed I am at times of my white hair and wrinkled hands—my hands!—or my neck. My God! In a few weeks I'll turn 86.

And then I'm ashamed of being ashamed. Yet deep in my unconscious lies the unvoiced certainty that age means rejection, that ancient women are killed as witches or stoned from the tribe, wandering in the wilderness. I know it's not true, but somehow the myth prevails.

Eighty-six feels so much older than 85, even though I'll never be this young again.

This week my daughter Molly, knowing my love of theater, took me to Boston for an early birthday present to see the high-tech deconstruction performance of Chekov's *The Cherry Orchard*, directed by the Ukrainian artist Igor

Golyak, with the dancer Baryshnikov playing the ancient servant, Firs. (Gosh! What a gift!)

Then there was more.

Before the performance, I asked to stop at CVS for cough drops. (What's worse than trying not to cough in a performance?) I dashed into a nearby store, hurrying lest I keep my daughter waiting, the car still running. I found the right aisle, snatched a bag of cough drops, and, hurrying to the checkout line, bumped so hard into someone that it jolted us both. I turned toward the brown wool coat visible out of the corner of my eye—"Oh, I'm sorry"—and met the sharp, reproving eyes of a dark-skinned woman, perhaps in her 40s. She frowned so piercingly that for a moment I thought she was going to hit me.

I reached out one hand: "I'm so sorry. Forgive me." Then I turned back to the checkout, only to hear her call after me.

"You are so beautiful," she said, and repeated it. "You are so beautiful! The way you hold yourself. The way you are dressed. You are a princess. You are so beautiful."

I was stunned.

For suddenly I saw that she was the one who was beautiful, with her dark coloring and high cheekbones, an Egyptian princess in a worn brown coat too big for her.

"No, you are," I called.

We stood immobile, staring at one another and smiling, smiling. In that moment, time stopped. I felt as if I were being shown something important. As if I'd never seen before. Is everyone so beautiful? I moved away to pay for my cough drops, but I was shaken by the encounter and by the intimacy of that moment—and also uplifted. Me, beautiful? At 85, almost 86, I'm beautiful?

But what about the mirror? What about my inner critical judge?

I feel better writing this out loud to you, when today I feel old again and in need of the compliment. She came like an angel to speak what I needed to hear at that moment. And to show me herself as well—how beautiful she was when I could see into her core. Clearly, it's time to consider my mother's words: look harder, dive deeper, listen more acutely. Try to See.

If there's anything I learn as I get older, it's that I still lug around that nagging, critical inner voice. She's trying to protect me with news I've failed. I wish instead of pushing down the voice, I could welcome her instead: "Oh, it's You again. Come in. Tell me your troubles. Let's have a cup of tea."

Why do I find my friends at this age beautiful but cannot see it in myself?

Meanwhile, I am once again smiling with my Beloved, the Universe (as I call God), who sent me this sweet birthday present. Years ago, I had an African American friend who became a pastor, the kind who knew chapter and verse of every biblical reference and whose voice lilted with praise even in ordinary conversation. One day when I felt discouraged and telephoned her, she told me how she wakes up every morning and says, "OK, Husband. What do you want to do today? What fun thing have you thought up for us to do?"

She didn't mean her husband, Dickie, snoring beside her in bed, but her true husband, the God of her understanding, who was her best friend and also sister, mother, father, and secret lover.

I've never forgotten the joy in her voice as she told me of her love. And of her anticipation of each day: "OK, Husband, what fun are we going to have today?"

Is Love Different at This Age?

November 14

Dear Eleanor,

Thanksgiving rolling round again and I've been thinking about gratitude. Someone said to me the other day, "You're so positive. It's easy to see your glass is half full."

I broke out laughing. "My glass is full to overflowing," I answered, "spilling over, running down, boundless abundance."

I think the Universe loves to be thanked. I think when we are conscious of the gifts poured on us, the Universe turns itself inside out to give us more. Sometimes I receive things I've forgotten even wanting years before (like the remote garage door opener)—and suddenly I find I have it, just a little gift, a little love note handed out.

But the greatest of all is this mystery of love.

Do you, at 59, wonder who you are? I do. Am I different now, as an old woman, from earlier in my life? I'm still me, with all my flaws and failings, and not even my ideas are much different from any I had before. I'm neither smarter nor dumber, although my thoughts, like my feet, move slower now, and sometimes a name or word will suddenly go walkabout and just as mysteriously appear again, with a triumphant little two-step: ta-DA!

But thirty years later, it's easier to let things go. I've learned I'm not in control of anyone. Or anything. Not the politicians, not the car that died today (battery), or the printer that has a mind of its own. As a consequence, I find myself with a degree of equanimity that I don't remember earlier. I don't fall into such labile moods as earlier in my life. There's an old Sufi story of the Persian sage meditating near some whirling dervishes. A student asks, "Doesn't it bother you, all that noise and activity happening right next to you?" And he answered, "I just let them whirl."

A more important question might be: is love different at age 85 from love in my 20s or 30s or 50s or 60s? I could argue that my love now runs quieter, deeper, stronger. It is the profound dark waters of the Pacific Trench instead of the glistening, light-shattered surface of ocean waves.

But is that true?

Here's a curious fact: I never fell in love until I was in my 20s—and that was with the man I married, David. I never had a teenage crush. But as I've traveled through the years, I find that love—and I mean erotic and passionate love—has hit with increasing frequency. The older I am, the more I love. And un-possessively. Isn't that odd?

I remember hearing about one gentleman of 96 who fell in love with a 91-year-old woman in the same nursing facility, and she with him. Then the woman's daughter moved her mother to live closer to her in New Jersey, and it didn't matter that the mother was in love with the old man. She was snatched away, kidnapped without power to protest.

It's a cliché to say it broke his heart. He stormed in grief, convinced she had left him for another man.

The older I get, the more I meet people, the more convinced I am that we must only work on ourselves, to grow in grace. The only thing we can do about people is to love them.

—Dorothy Day, *All the Way to Heaven, Selected Letters*

So what do I have to say about love in later years? I grow silent before its majesty. Love springs up constantly, at every age, like desert grass in rain. It attacks you suddenly, unexpectedly, the arrows of Eros, and it delivers always a heart-lifting surge of joy and creativity, the inexorable, desperate, painful uncertainty, longing, helplessness, tears, torture, and release.

I remember when I was in my 50s asking my dear friend Dorothy Clarke, then in her 90s, whether she still felt sexual desire.

"Oh yes," she answered. "The other night I had such a beautiful dream. . . ." Her eyes took on a glow, her face shining. "I think it's there until you die."

It's the life-force energy that George Bernard Shaw wrote of.

Once I interviewed the Dalai Lama. I asked, "Were you ever sorry that you were chosen as a child for this position?"

He answered, "No."

"Hmm," I murmured thoughtfully. "No desire."

"Oh, I have desire," he interrupted quickly. "In my dreams I often dream of violence and of sexual things. But even in dreams, I remember I am a Buddhist monk. And," he continued with a gentle smile, "my monkhood is the dearest to my heart."

*Those who love deeply never grow old;
they may die of old age, but they die young.*
—Arthur Wing Pinero, *The Princess and the Butterfly*, 1897 play

I think we are formed of love. The very cells of our bodies are made of love—as are those of trees and dogs and horses and wildlife and weasels and the upthrusting urgent tulip-growth, thundering through the soil, everything demanding life, operatic love: this whole remarkable living earth. I think the soul, if you will, our very essence, is simply Love, shining with goodness, kindness, innocence, hope, intelligence in an overflowing, boundless, endless outpouring of Love. Maybe that's what we finally learn with age—what we knew when we were 5—and forgot in all the frenzy of living. We forgot that even pain and rage and violence are only our ignorant distorted efforts to reach the safety of love.

(What crap, says the snarky side of me: if we're made of love, we sure cover it over well with the concrete, mud, and filth of hate, rape, violation, and other efforts of our souls.) (Oh, do be quiet, you.)

How do we reconnect with it? Meditation helps. Walking. Sitting in the woods or standing beside ocean waters, watching the ceaseless breakers throw themselves onto the beach, clawing, clutching at the land. Wherever we find ourselves resting in stillness. Stillness is how we remember to stoke the inner fires where the soul shines out, asking nothing in return.

In these older years, with the luxury of no longer working for a living, with the shedding and simplifying of desires, I think I begin the great adventure of finally Being Alive.

It is best as one grows older to strip oneself of possessions, to shed oneself downward like a tree, to be almost wholly earth before one dies.
—Sylvia Townsend Warner, *Lolly Willowes*

But, oh, Eleanor, no sooner do I crow about this than I am felled by humility. I have enough money to live on. What of those who live in poverty? Hundreds of thousands in our country are homeless, living on the streets or in boxes. Thirteen percent of our population—44 million people—go hungry every day, little children without food. (And around the world it is 10 percent, or 800 million, who go hungry every day.) What courage they show! What of those bombed out of their homes in war, or victims of fire, flood, famine, earthquakes, tsunamis, mudslides? I am ashamed to talk of love when all that is really needed is money. I boast how easy it is in old age to "let go"—what hypocrisy! What *lies* I tell myself!

Oh, brave humanity. I am in awe.

Coming Back

December 1

Dear Eleanor,

Last night I dreamed about my childhood friend Kitty
Cromwell. Eleanor, you are a filmmaker. Imagine Kitty
as a little girl, with fire-red hair, straight as taut string,
and her awkward, jerking gait, her eyes bulging behind
thick glasses. She knew she was ugly. She was told it often
enough. She knew she was stupid. That, too, she was told.
When we children wanted a playdate, either at her house
or mine, we could not go out, by proclamation of her
mother, unless Kitty had scrubbed the kitchen (with me
helping)—yet the family kept a live-in cook and one
or two maids.

I think her mother took a special dislike to Kitty, her
fifth and final child. She had trained as a concert pianist
before marriage finished off that idea. (In those long-ago
1940s and '50s, a woman's career, especially if Catholic,
was "wife.") Kitty's mother spent her day on a chaise in her
bedroom, resting, and we children tiptoed carefully round
the house lest she be disturbed.

57

Nonetheless, Kitty inherited her remarkable musical gift. Kitty could play anything by ear. One day she was re-creating a Beethoven sonata on the piano that she'd heard her mother playing earlier, when the doorbell rang. Instantly, Kitty stopped. She knew enough to stop. Her mother opened the door to her friend, who cried, "Oh, Maria, I heard you playing just now. It was the best I've ever heard you play!" Kitty was forbidden to touch the piano for weeks. She was never given music lessons, never taught to read music, never encouraged. What she learned early was that she was stupid, ugly, and unacceptable. Looking back, I think her mother was mentally ill, or high on Valium, or both, but those were concepts we children could not have imagined.

Later, Kitty broke with her family, moved to North Carolina, and became a spiritual recluse. She married in late life, only to find her husband had dementia. She took care of him until he died.

Poor Kitty. My lifelong friend. She died five or six years ago.

You will come to know things that can only be known with the wisdom of age and the grace of years. Most of those things will have to do with forgiveness.
—Cheryl Strayed, *Tiny Beautiful Things: Advice on Love and Life from Dear Sugar*

In my dream Kitty came to me. In the dream she was dead, and she was smiling and smiling at me. She still had flaming red hair, but her movements were easy, graceful, and she was beautiful. She was ecstatic.

"I'm coming back," she told me. "I can come back now." Meaning, I think, that she had earned the right to have another life. And all around her stood a crowd of people cheering her on.

I woke up happy.

I think the news is real. I'm so glad. Yet I marvel that after that one life she would dare to try another.

Ten days ago, I wrote you about my hurt and anger and dislike of Caroline. Yesterday, walking together, she began to talk intimately about her unhappy childhood and the difficulties of caring for her mother, who at 90 had come to stay in her tiny apartment: her dreams of writing destroyed, her life taking a path she hadn't planned.

I haven't remembered to pray for her more than two or three times—and suddenly, as if she's a different person, I like her.

How is it that I'm still learning the same lessons over and over, given the same lessons again and again? Be vulnerable. Be open. Stop pretending in good WASP fashion that everything is fine.

There's no one to dislike. All I need to do is to look deeper. Everyone is struggling. Everyone is hurting. Will I ever learn? It's just forgive, forgive, forgive.

Oh, Eleanor, I love you so much. Look what you are doing for me, just by giving me this chance to consider these things. I love writing to you, even if I never send these letters. I think of you moving about your beautiful apartment in Paris, or striding forcefully down the streets, nodding to the shop-keepers you know, or holding important meetings with other film producers, or dashing off to Senegal, where you have a whole other life that I have never seen, or flying to America. It all seems so exotic.

And now I must rush to market. All I do is run small errands. And see doctors. (Lucky me, I have doctors!)

With love,
Sophy

All the Lives We Live

Dearest Eleanor,

One of the things that happens with the luxury of time is that you get to relive your stories, your memories, reading new insights into them. My mind is a time machine.

I can't stop thinking about your grandmother, my Aunt Eleanor, after whom you were named. When we were children, she terrified us, so fixed were her ideas on how things ought to be. God help us children if we used the wrong fork, slumped in our chairs, interrupted when in adult company. My two first cousins—Charlie, your father, and Vicky, his sister—had a rough time of it. Their father, the Admiral, accustomed to military obedience, had schooled himself never to show emotion, and Aunt Eleanor followed suit, although she was by nature creative, playful, full of spirit. Uncle Bev once told me that if a cannon went off at his back, he would only slowly turn. He wanted never to show surprise or fear. Or vulnerability, I suppose.

The only rebellion I ever saw from either of my cousins lay in calling their father by his first name, instead of

Daddy or Dad. Neither did I ever discover what this informality implied.

We were all in love with Charlie, your father, the only boy in three generations. After college, he went into the Marines to prove that he could be a "man." He hated it. Years later, dying of brain cancer, he told me that he was still angry with his father for the rules he'd been forced to follow. Charlie was by nature as gentle and thoughtful a man as you could meet. Killing didn't suit him. I will never forget the day out at Gaga's farm when Charlie, then 12 and stalking proudly up and down the lawn with his new BB gun, lifted the gun now and then to his shoulder to aim. "Pow." I was 5 or 6, I suppose, trotting after him, admiring.

Then he shot a robin. It fell to the ground. I covered my mouth with both hands in my dismay, and he was as horrified as I.

"You must never tell anyone," he admonished me, and I nodded. Of course I wouldn't tell. It was one of the worst things you could do in all the world—to shoot a bird, or cut a tree branch, or disturb the bees in our grandfather's hives in the orchard. It was as bad as making noise when the grown-ups were talking. We buried the bird secretly. Charlie dragged home, all delight in his new gun dimmed.

He married your mother, whose family for generations seemed so intertwined with ours that I could never unravel the tangles. And you were born, and then your siblings. Aunt Eleanor was especially proud of you, her first grandchild and her namesake. But she was still fiercely rule bound, still determined to follow all the unspoken injunctions and make sure that we youngsters made no mistakes. . . . I understand only now how filled with anxiety she must have been, a walking beehive, trying to toe the line herself.

The great thing about getting older is that you don't lose all the other ages you've been.
—Madeline L'Engle

Do you remember how, when you wrote your grandmother a thank-you letter, she would return it to you marked with red corrections? She wanted to be a writer, and, like all the girls of her Southern upbringing, she was not offered college, never allowed the freedom given to men. Late in life, she self-published two books. And who knows what courage it took for her to put herself forth like that? I find myself bowing to her in my imagination for taking writing classes in her 60s at American University, for daring to express and reveal herself.

But that happened only after.

After the death of both her children a few months apart, Charlie from a brain tumor and Vicky from a fall from a horse.

A few months later, my husband's sister, who worked as the children's librarian at Potomac School (first through eighth grade) where Vicky's children attended, told me that at Grandparent's Day, she had come across Uncle Bev, the Admiral, alone in the library. He was sitting in a tiny tot-chair, tears running down his face. She backed out quietly, unseen.

(I told this story to an Italian American friend, who cried: "She backed out?! She didn't go sit beside him and take his hand? She didn't comfort him? Oh, you WASPs! I can't believe you!")

My parents spoke with admiration of how your grandmother behaved with the strength of a Roman matron at Vicky's funeral, all smiles, evidencing no grief. I remember her catching my arm outside the church to introduce me to a friend. "Oh, Sophy, I want you to meet Mrs. Smith." From my present vantage point, I no longer see a Roman matron but a woman so broken that only the habit of manners remained.

After that she changed. Life has a way of bringing us to our knees. After that, nothing that had ruled felt important anymore, not the right fork, not the repression of anger, not the rebellious thought. She had cracked open.

And out of her pain poured love.

I wake up at two in the morning sometimes, and, lying vulnerable in the dark, I toss, turn, cringe with horror, regret, and remorse for things done and things not done, my sins of commission and omission. There's no way in the world to make up. Everyone is dead. Curiously, it is usually the omissions—the things I didn't do—that keep me awake.

Perhaps this is another gift of age: that we are given the time to reexamine and relive the past, this time from a wider perspective. We are given the chance to be open to the wildness, the ferocity, the magnificence of it all. And to make amends, if not to them, then forward to someone now living who needs a moment of deep listening, or forgiveness, or the nod of understanding: our pathetic attempt to make up for the selfishness and stupidity and ignorance of youth.

I have the impression, looking back, that everything makes sense. What started as a hopeless mass of unconnected congeries appears, in hindsight, to have held a narrative, and the narrative is all about letting go instead of being jailed by fear. I'm not the only octogenarian to discover this.

"After twenty or thirty years," said one friend, "you realize things worked out better than you thought. The job you didn't take . . . the person you refused . . ."

We need unlimited forgiveness, especially of ourselves. Being a human is hard.

Am I wandering in these musings?

I feel I'm groping for what I want to say. It's just out of reach, something important. To pass along.

Age has given me what I was looking for my entire life—it has given me me. I fit into me now. I have an organic life, finally, not necessarily the one people imagined for me, or tried to get me to have. I have the life I longed for. I have become the woman I hardly dared imagine I would be.

—Anne Lamott, *Plan B: Further Thoughts on Faith*

My Aunt Eleanor died at 88 and Uncle Bev at 91. They had both moved into a retirement home, and I'm ashamed now that I offered no help with their move or with the disposition of antiques and family treasures that went back generations. By then I'd half fallen in love with Uncle Bev, kind, generous—and so handsome! His sparkling eyes. Even in his 80s he stood tall and straight. As for Aunt Eleanor, your grandmother, you understand that by then I adored her. With the deaths of Charlie and Vicky, she was no longer the ferocious aunt of my childhood. We talked a lot about death, about the aura of light that I see surrounding people, even about the Hereafter, which I have been graced to glimpse. Unlike her sisters, Aunt Eleanor abhorred church. I'd call her a Freethinker. She listened, amused, when I talked about the light, or about alternative healing modalities, or about angels, but she didn't believe me for a minute.

And then one day she phoned me. She had something to tell me. Could I come visit? I flew to her hospital bed. She told me she had had a dream and, in the dream, she stood at a river, and on the other side a crowd of friends were all calling and waving to her. She wanted to cross the river— everything was light struck, streaming with light—and when she woke up, she knew beyond any doubt that dying was going to be all right.

"You were right," she said again and again, holding my hand, patting my hand, as she lay back on her pillow. Her eyes were shining. And I could see that she had let go of everything that stood in the way of her being who she really was.

In my mind, we are climbing a staircase that winds inside a tower of glass. From every step we see the landscape outside the windows, mountains, valleys, rivers, lakes, and seas. The stairwell winds round and round inside the glass walls, and we climb (or sometimes descend a step or two), each level offering a different view of the same external land.

What we are looking at is our internal life, past and present, our place on this strange planet of suffering and redemption.

In aging, we see at different and higher viewpoints while we climb upward, round and round.

When Is Old?

Dear Eleanor,

When I was 10, I thought a girl of 15 was "old." I remember at 23 snickering at my grandmother for calling a man of 40 "a nice young man." That's because anyone older than you is "old."

My daughter Molly teaches writing at the University of Massachusetts. The other day she asked her class of 19- to 21-year-olds to bring in a page they had written to read. One student brought the cover letter for his job application for an internship in the Massachusetts attorney general's office, competing against hundreds of applicants.

He began to read:

"Dear Meghan—"

Molly stopped him. "Do you know Meghan?" she inquired.

"No, but I want her to know who I am."

Molly thought a moment. "Is this a formal office? Informal? What will you be wearing in the job?"

"Oh, I'll wear a suit and tie."

"So it's formal. . . . I think maybe you might want to use a formal form of address. You don't know her yet."

"But I want her to know me for whom I am."

"Well, you can do that in the body of the letter, can't you?"

One of the other students piped up. "No, I think he's right. I had a job with a law firm, and I called everyone Mr. Jones, or Ms. Jones, and they all said, 'Call me John,' or 'Call me Zoe.' So I think he can address her as Meghan."

"But they gave you permission," said Molly. "Isn't this different?"

A lively discussion ensued, with the class mostly siding with the student, until one young man in the back raised his hand.

"I think Molly's right," he said, calling his teacher by her first name, as she had asked them to do. "I think you should change it."

"Yes, but Molly's an older generation!" cried another.

So it is that we slip invisibly from one age to the next. To me, she's a lovely young woman, and to the students, she's "old."

Cousin Phyllis was my mother's first cousin, a spunky, active spinster in her 90s when she fell and broke her hip. She was placed in an old person's home in Washington, D.C., a gloomy stone fortress dating back to the Civil War that still carried, carved into the stone over the doorway, its ruthless name: "Home for the Incurables."

It was a horrible place, filled with long tiled corridors where the aged in wheelchairs plucked at a blanket across their laps as they waited in the empty halls for visitors who did not come. They had no distractions apart from a tiny TV in their bedrooms. Cousin Phyllis was the daughter of my grandfather's brother—not the crazy artist who became addicted to opium but the brother who had served all his life as Episcopal rector of the Church of the Epiphany on New York Avenue in Washington, D.C. Cousin Phyllis was a Good Christian. She served her father's church her whole life long. But when she was put into the Home, her pretty little apartment was dismembered, her own possessions gone, and when I (a young mother at the time) took her out occasionally for ice cream, her scorn and disgust for the others in the Home impressed me.

"They're OLD!" she would snarl with a disdainful curl of her lip. She hated every minute.

Who wouldn't?

"You have earned your crown in heaven," she would gush as she ate a hot fudge sundae on our outings or drove around Washington to see something besides the Incurables. "Your crown in heaven."

Oh, but she could be snarky, this Good Christian.

Her room had barely space for a bed and a vertical chest of drawers, on which a tiny TV crowded the black-and-white family photos. The window at her headboard took up the wall that faced the door. That's how small the room was: a contrast from the city mansion she had grown up in, with its carriage houses and view of the Potomac River.

For her 96th birthday I baked her a cake. I set it on the dresser, pushing aside the small photo of her father and a few faded relatives. She was thrilled to have me hand her a piece on a china plate with a silver fork. She sat on the edge of her bed to eat. I said something about having made the cake large enough to share with others on her corridor.

"I'm not going to share it with THEM!" she cried in horror. "They're OLD!"

It was hers, and she was not about to let it go, not when nothing was left to her anymore but memories.

And here, Eleanor, I must say something about Home. Sometimes your possessions are the only thing keeping you stable. I remember Aunt Kate, then 102, telephoning me at night.

"Sophy, I don't know what's happened. I don't know where I am. I want to go home."

She was having a sunset moment.

"Well, is your furniture there? The tables? Your pictures on the walls?"

"Yes. That's what's so strange. But it's not my house. I want to go home."

"That's really curious. Are you all right? Where are you now? Are you in bed?"

"Yes, I'm in bed."

"Well, it's really late. Listen, right now, just go to sleep. I'll come over in the morning and we can straighten this out. I'll take care of it in the morning."

In the morning, of course, rested, she knew herself again. But in that frightening moment, it was her furniture, her paintings, the rug on the floor that grounded her, that kept her safe.

This is why it's so hard to move an older person into assisted living. She can't find herself anymore. Our memories, gathered into our possessions, hold us in their arms.

"At what age are you old?" I asked a friend, Michele.

"When your parents die," she answered without hesitation. "When you move to the top of the ladder."

I'm not sure the response counts, since she is only in her late 60s.

"You are old when you decide you are," said another. "When it's too much trouble to pretend any longer and you just decide to stop coloring your hair or wearing makeup. 'Oh, what the heck,' you say."

"You are old when you start telling your age," Annette agreed, having spent her life knocking off the years. "Then you get to play the old card."

To AARP, old begins at age 50.

For Medicare, old (and receiving medical insurance) is 65.

Social Security dates old at 64.

When Social Security was started in 1935, the average age of death for white men at birth was 61, and for white women it was 65. For Blacks and other minorities, it was only 51 for men and 55 for women. In the 1930s, therefore, only a small percentage of the population survived long enough to receive large benefits.

Is "old" a projection? Or is it a perception?

Time

Dearest Eleanor,

Today I saw a woman get out of her car carrying a sack
of laundry—such a modest, unimportant sight, but I stopped
in mid-step, struck by how beautiful she was, this ordinary,
middle-aged, sagging woman, and by her act of fumbling
half out of the car. It took my breath away. For a fraction
of a second, time stopped. For a fraction of a second, I was
"seeing," truly. I think if a frame had been placed around the
car—the woman, one leg extended to the curb, her sack of
laundry—if that image hung framed in a museum, everyone
would pay to stand admiring it. If time could stop.

I don't have a clue what Time is. Of course, we all know
Einstein's classic formula, $E = mc^2$, in which he affirms
that Energy is Mass multiplied by Light (c) (traveling at an
unbelievable 186,000 miles/second) multiplied by itself, or
squared. But we are also informed that Light cannot exist
without Time. If Time were stopped, there'd be no Light.

Since Time can't be stopped, however, Light moves on at 607 million miles per hour, on and on. But why Light plays any part in Energy, much less so important as to be squared (Why squared? And how do you square Light anyway?), is all beyond my poor brain. What does Time have to do with Space? A communion so close we name it Space-Time now.

I know only that Time slides by, sometimes swiftly, sometimes slowly. Or perhaps it doesn't pass. Perhaps it merely circles round and round, as theoretical physicist Carlo Rovelli proposes, in some illusion that doesn't correspond to physical reality. To make Time more confusing, it has sped up as I've aged, fleeing now so fast that it seems I hardly throw my leg out of bed in the morning before it's nightfall and I'm crawling back in. I am on a train that in childhood went so slowly that one revolution of the wheels might take a season or year. In my teens it chuffed and clicked steadily along the tracks, and by my 40s it had opened up, moving smoothly through the fields and across the rivers, clickety-click. Now in my 80s I'm on the bullet train, with fields and cities sweeping past the windows in a blur. Time has increased in speed.

I remember my grandmother Gaga on her 80th birthday (an age to me incomprehensible, a millennium) murmuring, "It's all gone so fast."

At the same time, myself now more than 80, I find I have more time. I have time now to muse on things.

Time is a created thing. To say, "I don't have time," is like saying, "I don't want to."

—Lao Tzu

In 1964, when I was 28, my grandmother, lying under a blanket on a hot summer day, astonished me with the announcement that she had shaken the hand of a soldier who had fought at the Battle of Waterloo (1815). What?! Suddenly, 150 years collapsed into one handshake. In 2023, I can say that I kissed a man born before the Civil War. He was my grandfather, the Doctor, born in 1858, 166 years ago. The past is only a footstep away.

When my parents were born, in 1902 and 1909, respectively (more than one hundred years ago), legs or horses were the common form of transportation, and most people used oil lamps. My parents lived through the horrors of the First World War; the 1918 flu that killed 18 million, almost one-third of the world population; then the 1929 Crash and the Depression that left destitute men and women queuing in bread lines that ended only with the Second World War, itself rung in like clockwork only twenty years after the War to End All Wars. By the end of WWII, my parents were still only in their 30s or 40s. That war was followed by the atom bomb, the Cold War, fear, anxiety, recession, high gas prices, the Vietnam War, the Civil Rights movement, the Women's Movement, Watergate. They adjusted to the telephone, TV, high-speed cars on intercontinental highways, and commonplace plane travel. Both my parents died on the cusp of computers, instantaneous communication, and further catastrophes.

Yet despite the horrors, they were immeasurably happy. In my memory they are always roaring with laughter, dressing up for parties, utterly involved in their friends and lives. At the end, of course, challenged by cancer and strokes, things got hard. At the end they suffered cruelly.

I suspect that everyone does. At the end takes courage.

For me, at 86, this historical perspective colors my world. One friend mentioned over dinner that he's not concerned about everything going to hell, because it's always been going to hell—what the hell?

Is that equated with wisdom? I don't know. But I'm convinced that things have a way of working themselves out. Often for the better, or at least for the good. I refuse to worry. People are infinitely inventive. We'll find something still unheard of that will take care of political disasters, corrupt and unjust decisions, or even climate change—some new clean energy derived perhaps from tides and ocean waves, or plastics, or human trash. Perhaps from the sun and stars.

What we won't see is a change in human greed, fear, pride, arrogance, violence . . . or in our innate goodness, our altruistic kindness always warring with our fear.

As you ripen, you'll notice that time is the weirdest thing in the world, that surprises are relentless, and that getting older is not a stroll but an ambush.
—Andrew Solomon

Humans have only been on earth for a million years or so. Not all that many, when compared to the 4.5 billions years that the planet has been tirelessly circling its star, or the 5 billion more circling still to come before our sun explodes.

Back to the matter of age, though. We have the impression that you get numerically old and then everything goes downhill. Don't count on it, Eleanor. A lot of those old girls are wicked and not against pulling the "old card" as needed. One day, some years ago, a distant relative telephoned me to say that he would be in town on a particular date and,

having no car, wondered whether I could drive him to see
Aunt Kate, whom he had not seen in some years. And so I
did. I called Aunt Kate first to warn her of the visit, and on the
appointed day I picked him up at his hotel with all his baggage
to visit her before ferrying him to his plane back home. He
was well into his 60s, long, lean, a little bowed forward by the
weight of life. Once settled in the car:

"How is she?" he murmured in a doleful voice.

"Oh, she's fine," I said chirpily. "She's in a wheelchair now,
but you'll see: she's just as bright as a button." I don't know
whether he was relieved or disappointed.

And so we drove merrily on.

At the retirement home, we passed through the generous,
elegant entry, took the elevator to her floor, and walked
down the well-carpeted neutral colors of the corridor to her
apartment door, where we knocked and were let in by her
part-time nurse.

"Hello, Aunt Kate. Look who I've brought—"

To my surprise, Aunt Kate, in her wheelchair, hardly
glanced up from a small pile of letters and greeting cards
on the table beside her. She picked one up, ignoring us, and
examined it as if she'd never seen a card before.

I reminded her of the name of her visitor as we tend to do
with the older generation, in case they don't remember names.
She nodded with regal attention and offered us a cup of tea

(spoken in three syllables in her lovely Southern accent, a "cu-u-up"). But that done, she paid no more attention to us, instead muttering with her papers or staring for minutes at the wall. I won't say that she drooled, but she slumped and tilted in her wheelchair until the nurse came to pull her upright again. She neither spoke nor responded to this distant relative, and when we left, I was as shaken as he.

"I guess she has bad days," I said, having never seen her like this before. We drove in silence to the airport.

That would have been the end, except that a week later I was again at her apartment, where I found her this time her usual active, chipper self. A friend knocked while I was there and entered, welcomed in with Aunt Kate's utter delight.

"You won't believe who came to see me two days ago," she announced before her friend had hardly stepped across the threshold. She pronounced his name.

"No!"

"Yes. Well, I just pretended to be goo-goo-ga-ga. I wasn't about to speak to him! I can't believe he dared to visit me! Wanting to inherit, I dare say, when I die."

"Well, let him dream," agreed her friend.

Of course, I wanted the whole story, which they were happy to pass on: how he had offended, and worse—without recognizing his lack of ethical plinth. It's a shocking story that I will happily repeat. You can decide his guilt. He chose

to fly to New York for a ho-hum board meeting of the Metro-
politan Museum of Art over bidding goodbye to his dying
aunt. By the time he arrived in Virginia, she had died: she who
left him all her money, she who loved him as her own son.
Aunt Kate was not about to forgive.

The moral is: don't underestimate the very ancient.
They are sharper than you think. And memories last as
long as Time.

PART 2

Voices

Talking recently with a group of women my age, I asked them to name one word that described this period of their 80s. What's it like to be an octogenarian?

Freedom, said one.

Curious, said another.

Astonishing, said one woman who has just fallen head over heels in love with a man after losing her female partner of twenty-one years.

Awake. "I'm aware," said a woman only in her 70s, "in ways I never felt before, of how temporary everything is. Because of that, everything seems more—" She gave a wave of her hand, unable to find words for her depth of feeling.

Scared, responded one woman diagnosed with initial dementia. With the loss of words and the frightening sense of losing control, the world has become confusing.

Process, said Sarah, and then explained: "This is a time when you can't help but cast through memories, both yours and those of others, friends. The memories bring up humor, pathos, anguish, delight. Life is so deep now, especially for those of us who have been in analysis, or who purposefully meditate. I don't know how it is," she added humbly, "for those who haven't meditated."

Gratitude. "I dislike these one-word challenges. I never seem to find one that nails it. What about—'mega-opportunity for gratitude?'—for health, nearby family, friends, adequate finances. . . . I feel like a happy air plant thriving in a slowly shrinking terrarium. If such existed."

Acts of kindness, said one sprightly lady, happily offering three words. "People see me and immediately help me with groceries, open doors, give me a seat. Oh, so many little acts!"

Visibility. "I've been invisible all my life. All my life I suppressed myself. Now I'm not. Of course, whether I speak up depends on the community. But I don't want to live any longer in this prison of passivity, this 'I-can't-challenge.' . . . Why didn't I speak up earlier? It was my upbringing in an alcoholic house. It is only with ACOA meetings that I've started now to dare."

Liberation, said a woman of 87 who spends her time on the tennis court. "I don't care if I embarrass anyone," she said, echoing the friend who has released herself from inhibitions. She has moved to a retirement home and runs in a crowd fifteen years younger. "In assisted living, you end up dropping far-off friends. Or friends drop away. Or die. That's sad."

Beautiful. "This is the most beautiful time of my life," said Bunnie over breakfast. "Of course I have the Program," she

continued, meaning one of the twelve-step programs.
"I don't know what people who don't have that do. I've never
been closer to my Higher Power. I don't care what others
think of me. This is my time for ME. I have all these physical
problems, but I have learned compassion for myself."

Uncomfortable, responds one woman, tucking frightened
hands into her lap. "I'm in early-stage dementia. I'm forget-
ting things. It's upsetting. It's never happened to me before.
Losing my memory, I mean. I'm beginning to get involved
with psychology," she lifted her eyes, in appeal, courageous
in her struggle to adapt.

"I agree," piped up another, also diagnosed with early-
stage dementia. "How do you know where you're going?
That's my reality. I have my husband and my daughter with
me, and they do the best they can. I can still paint. My visual
memory is still good. But words . . ." She trailed off. Who
are we without our words? Without our stories? Without
thoughts? "I think, therefore I exist," wrote Descartes. What
if we lose our thoughts?

"I don't have a word," said another in the group,
and she rose to her feet, too distressed to stay seated on
the couch. "I work. I'm a lawyer. I can't retire. I keep
thinking about retiring, but I don't do it. I can't." Panic
might be her word. There is panic in her voice. And why
not, when millions are homeless, when 13 percent of the

population—43 million people—goes hungry in the United States every day?

I am reminded of a friend in Washington, similarly strapped financially, who worked in real estate well into her 90s. She, too, would have loved to quit earlier and finally managed it at 92, living on Social Security and savings.

Friendships, offered Dottie, a woman of 97. "It's difficult to settle on one word, but certainly friendships and compassion for others rank near the top." She lives in an assisted-living facility, with opportunity for social interaction. "I don't know what I'd do without my friends." She went on to proclaim that she doesn't feel more than 70 and finds that nearly everyone she meets is friendly and helpful. She is amazed to have lived so long and to be still learning at her age.

She is not afraid of death.

But not everyone finds their 80s happy. One woman (almost all my friends are women now) is pessimistic.

"Slower," she responded, then added, "No, there's nothing wonderful about these years." She finds walking difficult. She often experiences ageism, which comes, she says, primarily from the expectation of others that she doesn't know what she's doing. (I, too, find it annoying when my daughters assume I need help with something I'm perfectly capable of, or start to tell me how to live, as if I don't have twenty-five years' more experience than they—before I catch myself, delighted to see them so certain and so frightened for me. Aren't they beautiful to behold?)

A friend, now in assisted living, though not yet needing help, is not the only one my age to find this fast-paced period of change and technology confusing and complicated.

She finds love with family, friends, and church. She writes for joy but feels no new purpose or wisdom has come to her in these years. Indeed, she says she is lonelier now than in earlier years.

And no, if there is freedom and liberation, she has not experienced it. Age to her is suffocating.

In contrast Becky, at the opposite extreme, experiences liberation in being free to love her new man. "Falling in love, that's wonderful. I'm surprised by my robust- ness. I love this age! I can't fit all my answers into this small page."

She finds purpose: it is "to receive and transmit love and joy; to protect the planet's remaining green spaces; to listen and support younger climate activists; to develop relationships and support working women of another color and class; to expand my consciousness."

This sample of my circle is so small as to have no statistical meaning. The surprise, though, is how many—most—are upbeat, optimistic, full of vim and curiosity.

"As long as my health holds out," said one, not finishing her sentence. "I have committees, book clubs, curiosity, enthusiasm. . . ."

"What is there to be afraid of?" another said, laughing.

For happiness, we all agreed that having a community is important.

"Merely expressing yourself, and having a community in which to do it, is empowering. It releases energy. So, that is important to seek out in these later years."

And, also important, I would add, is to cultivate a few true, intimate friends to whom you reveal yourself totally, friends who are still curious, engaged, who seek out joy.

Acknowledging your age is also freeing, we agreed.

"There is something wonderful about being 'old,'" says Nan in Florida. "I am understanding the unfolding of my life so far, that is, from childhood to old age. Watching myself. I also find so much kindness from strangers."

"I thought I was old at 30," said one woman, "and again at 45. I never talked about my age. I wanted to be younger. If someone asked my age, I lied. I thought they were prying. When AARP told me when I reached 50 that I could now join the ranks of the old, I was appalled. Insulted. Then at 59 I was teaching English to Buddhist monks who acted differently to me. They treated me with respect. It changed my attitude."

"And what is wrong," I asked, "with being old?"

The question elicited a burst of laughter from one group, for everyone knew what was wrong: the daily reminders of the aging body—bowels, bladder, dry skin, eyes, ears, voice, the loss of strength in hands or legs. We have glasses for eyes and hearing aids for ears, but loss of strength cannot be recovered. That's where we need the kindness of others, and there seems to be a surprising surplus of this.

I told you, Eleanor, how all my life I have hunted out an older woman as a role model, someone in her 80s or 90s. When I was in my 40s, I preened myself, proud of helping my neighbor, an old lady in her 90s who still lived alone in her house across the street. Her name was Dorothy Clarke. Little did I know the gifts would come all from her to me.

"Oh, Sophy," she announced one day when she was 92, "I've learned so much since I was 90! I've learned more since I was 90 than in all my life."

Yet her life had shrunk to one room. When she woke each morning, she carefully dressed in panties, bra, corset (imagine!), stockings, underslip, frock, and simple black low-heeled shoes. She brushed her colored hair and tottered from one chair-back to the doorway, moving shakily to the kitchen to eat one small yogurt for breakfast. Then she sat in her chair by a window for the day, reading heavy biographies with a magnifying glass, or watching TV, or flipping through the many magazines she subscribed to, always curious about fashions, news, and times.

Sometimes a whole day passed without her speaking to anyone, unless to order a food delivery on the phone. At night she went back to bed. She lived like a yogi in a cave. Yet here she was telling me, "I've learned more since I was 90 than in all my life."

By the time she died at 96 or 97, she was disappointed each morning to have awakened one more time. By then she was anxious to go, and, though believing in reincarnation, she wanted none of it.

"I'm never coming back," she declared. "I've had enough." She'd fight with God never to take on another life.

How different from Gloria Steinem, who as I write this sentence is 89 and hiking alone in Namibia. But then, she's not yet 98.

I find it interesting that not a single person mentioned loneliness.

Isn't that what we imagine when we think of "old"? A lonely individual, locked perhaps in a wheelchair, plucking a plaid blanket, someone isolated and without company at a time when all friends and family have died.

But being alone and being lonely are not the same. I have never been so lonely as in the swirling activity of a crowded, noisy Washington, D.C., cocktail party. The din is deafening, and I am lost.

Sorrowful Statistics

Dearest Eleanor,

    Your question about "old" has sent me off in new directions, including research (imagine—not only search but search again), and what I find is contradictory, confusing, compelling, and contrary to a lot of what I have always thought true. Would you like to know about your future? It involves the past, for Future, flying in, always lands on the heaving shoulders of history. Here are some things to know: Life expectancy in the United States, which since the 1930s had climbed (most were dead by the time they reached the Social Security age of 65), has plummeted since the highs of the 1950s. It's true that many of us are living to ripe old age and that money helps significantly with longevity, but according to the Centers for Disease Control and Prevention (CDC), the average life expectancy at birth in the U.S. has dropped even in the last few years from 77.1 years to 76.1. Girls live longer than boys, but look: in 2021 the average life expectancy among comparable countries was 82.4 years. If you live in Europe, you'll probably stay alive six years longer than in the United States.

You, Eleanor, have a better chance of living a long time than an infant born today in the U.S., and lucky you, for living in France—because it gets worse.

I don't want to be a downer, but since the 1950s (says one study I found), fifty-six (!) countries have surpassed the U.S. in life expectancy. The numbers depend on which study you read, but it feels like a hawk tumbling from the sky. By 1968, the U.S. had fallen from twelfth in the world for longevity to twenty-ninth, and by 2023, it had collapsed to forty-third. What!? People in forty-three countries live longer than us?

No, maybe that's not right. Another study ranks the good old U.S.A. not forty-third but **sixty-first out of 237 nations**. No matter the ranking, the U.S. has the lowest life expectancy of any of the large wealthy countries, though we outspend everyone on health care.

At this point in my investigations, Eleanor, I had to stop and breathe. I felt faint. My beautiful country that I've believed in all my life has worse health care than China, Chile, Cuba, Albania, and of course the EU countries. . . . I had to close the computer, take a walk, stop thinking about it. It has taken me a few days to return to my research and find more comforting figures.

So here's the good news—or maybe not good at all: it turns out life expectancy in the U.S. is unevenly distributed. "More Americans die younger," states the *American Journal of Public Health* in June of 2023, "in states with conservative policies." Does that mean conservative politics? Conservative politicians? Republicans? I really don't want to know this.

While white males may expect to live to 71, Native American men have a life expectancy of only 61.5 years— shorter than men in India or Egypt. This doesn't mean that some don't live longer, but, good grief! I've already lived, Eleanor, more than twenty years longer than the average Native American male can expect to live today.

Have you ever found yourself compelled to keep on reading things you hate? Like Bluebeard's wife, I can't stop now that I've started opening the castle doors. I'm only telling you the tip of the iceberg, Eleanor, because my heart is twisting like a rag in my breast. The U.S. allows 22 maternal deaths per 100,000 births, and for Black women the figure is a stunning 49.5 maternal deaths per 100,000 live births. By comparison, Norway has . . . ZERO!

You're too young to have marched for women's rights in the late '60s and '70s. We were marching (never bra burning, by the way—that's made-up male media fodder: that never happened) and fighting for equal pay and the chance to experience life beyond broodmare. It never occurred to us to march for maternity care or the life of our babies. Nor did it occur to us to wonder why women live longer than men. Everyone knew this. It was common knowledge in my youth, factual as folk. Men burn out faster than women. I remember my mother, no feminist, sneering that men are weak. Which is why women have to serve them. Her other judgment, delivered in similar disgust: "Men are goats." Though whether she was referring to their smell or the faithless philandering of a neighbor, we children never learned.

Men die younger than women. But the figures are weird. More men die of diabetes in America than women do. More men die of cancer than women do. Boy babies die more often than girl babies. Adult men may die younger because they indulge in danger: guns, fast cars, smoking, alcohol, violence, drug abuse. But what does it mean that men commit suicide at higher rates than women? Or that boys are the ones to shoot up schools? What is going on?

I remember interviewing Margaret Mead once for an article on the Women's Movement. She told me our feminist cause would have no effect. Things might change, she said, but men will always be considered the more valuable. She told me that in every culture the work of men is considered more important than that of women. And this is true around the world. If the work of men lies in agriculture and cultivating the fields while women weave, then agriculture is given more value than weaving; if women till the fields while men are the ones to weave, then weaving is more highly valued. She continued that even if women broke into a male-dominated field, that field would soon lose value: it would become women's work.

I've thought about this a lot over the years. I've watched it in publishing, or nursing, or teaching, where men once dominated and where it soon became low-paid women's work, men leaving that field of battle for more profitable fights.

It is no surprise, then, that most medical and pharmacological studies are done on men.

I've gone off on another tangent, haven't I? But, Eleanor, guess what? Guess. It's ironic.

Despite our current interest in aging (actually in living longer; little interest in aging), we find almost no pharmacological studies of the elderly. Many of the trials had arbitrary age limits. I won't bore you with details, but in 839 trials to study drugs for heart disease, 53 percent excluded the elderly. Isn't that perfect? Who else gets heart disease?

Of course the studies don't include the elderly and aged. No point wasting money learning about aging from us! We're going to die. So both women and the elderly are deliberately excluded from most clinical trials. It makes me so mad I could stamp my foot like Rumpelstiltskin and rip myself in two!

And then I remember to laugh. The world goes round.

Meanwhile, more people are living into their 90s and 100s than ever before. Especially in Asia and Japan.

Oh dear. You can see where this is leading.

It's actually a real problem, Eleanor, that we have never seen before. In Japan, 800,000 fewer babies are born each year than the year before. Also in Japan, 450 schools close every year because of lack of children. The aging population is working well into their 60s and 70s. In the United States, despite more Americans living into their 80s, 90s, and 100s, in half the country more people are dying than are being born!

This is so disconcerting that Yusuke Narita, an assistant professor of economics at Yale, wrote a paper recently, taunting that the "elderly problem" in Japan's rapidly aging society could be resolved by the ancient practice of *seppuku*, or voluntary suicide, which would take care of a country with a low birth rate, the highest public debt in the developed world, and ever-expanding pension obligations. This chilling abstract designed to jump-start a conversation created an uproar of horror and disapproval.

But why?

I remember my father talking about one of his cases. He was defending an Eskimo man who lived in the most remote Arctic regions of Alaska and who had been charged with murder for putting his aged grandmother, according to time-honored tradition, out on the ice to die.

The question: Was her death justified to save the entire family? If she could not chew any longer, if the family had insufficient food to feed everyone, if she was already dying . . .? What was the moral and ethical thing to do? Save one life or save a larger group? And do the Anglo-American laws of the

Lower Forty-Eight supplant the ancient values and customs of that harsh environment?

My father won the case.

I don't know how I feel about this, Eleanor, but it's something that as a culture, as a country, we need to talk about. In 2024, 4.2 million Americans turned 65, 11,200 per day. By 2034, there will be more Americans past the retirement age of 65 than newborns.

For many, aging is going to be, if it isn't already, frightening and challenging, and I see no reason why we should not be discussing all possible solutions to a coming challenge. One solution might be to encourage immigration, a young and healthy population paying taxes to support us aged ones.

Why not?

Another solution, besides *seppuku*, might be for the federal government (which is to say, us, the people, gathered in discussion in community) to provide resources, as other developing nations do, to encourage families to have children and, once born, to provide them with maternal and child care, as other countries do, with food and medical assistance, education, mental health, clean air and water, and lead-free pipes.

My list could go on and on.

Where would the money come from to support this aging population (of voters)? One idea is to cut back funding for war, since the full U.S. military budget is already larger than that of the rest of the world's 144 nations combined. The only losers would be the arms manufacturers, and surely they could find other occupations, perhaps with federal training and assistance leading to work in AI, perhaps, or even in distributing care or helping to create health.

But I'm told that's simplistic.

Of course it's simple.

Good ideas always are.

PART 3

Love and Passion

Dearest Eleanor,

I said earlier I'd write about sex, but instead I want to talk of passion

Isabel Allende, when only 71, gave a TED Talk that you can view on YouTube called "How to Live Passionately—No Matter Your Age." According to the dictionary, passion is defined as: 1) a strong, barely controllable emotion, as in, "a person of impetuous passion," —2) an outburst of strong emotion, as in, "an orator who works himself into a passion," —3) an intense desire or enthusiasm for something, —4) intimate sexual love, "their all-consuming passion." Passion also means: 5) the suffering and death of Christ.

Her talk may have been given the title by the TED organization, for Allende was too smart to limit herself to "barely controllable emotions," which are not the first words that pop into mind when describing your 80s. But she speaks brilliantly of the freedom acquired in this period of life, how you shuffle off ancient grudges and resentments. You just don't have time to make yourself miserable with righteous indignation. You cast off vanity and ambition, the mistaken idea that accomplishment and achievements lead to admiration or will fill the empty hole at the heart. She mentions the wisdom of this age.

Allende encourages the softening of being open and vulnerable. Vulnerability is not a weakness, she says, but a sign of strength. She uses the word "mindfulness." Finally, she notices the presence of Death hovering nearby with its gift of spirituality.

But what she never talks about is passion. Or the passion of sexuality.

I know a couple in their mid-90s who still have a satisfactory sex life. It may not be as athletic as earlier, but it demonstrates desire carried into loving moderation. I know we never lose our sexual desire. I told you earlier about how I asked my beloved Dorothy Clarke, then in her mid-90s, whether she still felt sexual desire, and her answer (I was only a young and ignorant 42) startled me.

"Oh, Sophy," she said, her face lighting up, "I had the most wonderful dream last night about the most beautiful man. This man and me . . ." She said that you don't lose interest ever, not until you die. You may not be able to execute your desire, she said, but it's lurking there, the sign and symbol of our urgent life-force energy.

When I was in my 40s and 50s, I was surprised by how erotic and passionate I had become. Freed of the fear pregnancy (hysterectomy), I found that sensuality blossomed and bloomed in ways I could not have imagined earlier—certainly not in my 20s, when I still thought that anyone over 50 was plodding gravely toward the grave. Even my 70s were times of sensual passion—and satisfaction.

Now in my 80s I don't have a partner, and I want no more "barely controllable emotions," thank you. I can't imagine being penetrated, dry as my fluids are these days. My body is my own and not to be given away or shared. Which doesn't mean that I would turn away sweet cuddling if it came my way.

Epicurus, the Greek philosopher (341–270 B.C.E.) who dined most simply on bread, olives, and cheese—whose philosophy of virtuous simplicity became so corrupted into hedonist debauchery ("eat, drink, and be merry") that Dante threw him into the sixth circle of hell—pronounced that while pleasure is the touchstone of happiness, moderation alone leads to happiness. Simplicity doesn't mean you can't have an occasional feast or a blowout binge, but mostly you live without immoderate passions and the unfortunate consequences that so often follow.

It is impossible to live a pleasant life without living wisely and well and justly, and it is impossible to live wisely and well and justly without living a pleasant life.

—Epicurus. *Principles Doctrines*

A wealthy person without friends, freedom, or an examined life can never, he said, be happy, while one with friends, freedom, and the luxury of self-reflection is happy even without much money.

The mental pleasures of contemplation and friendships, he proposed, outweigh the physical ones of sex, wine, or the insatiable consumption of goods. For the former provides automatic satisfaction, while the latter leads only to further hunger and desire, longing and lack.

Basically, he's giving a commentary on our capitalistic culture, which exalts celebrity and consumption as a way to fill the empty hole at the heart that so many of us feel and that our culture seems to create. This emptiness can be filled, I have come to believe, only by a spiritual sense of who we really are—light-beings walking around encased in the concrete of physical form. To be completely happy, we need family, friends, a sense of service or meaning in life, a little money to live on, and from deep, deep within, a sense of connection to something greater than ourselves.

All this comes naturally to the octogenarian who sheds preoccupations as naturally as a snake sheds skin. Perhaps it explains the profound and steady happiness that almost everyone in my circle confessed. It certainly explains why huckstering advertising ignores us old hags. We have enough. We're living the Epicurean ideal, and we aren't buying anymore.

On the other hand, Eleanor, you are not yet even 60. These are wonderful years. As a woman, you hit the peak of your power. Go live! Eat it up. This is a time for passionate sexual desire and for throwing yourself furiously against obstacles in your work. Try. Succeed. Fail. And fail again. Test yourself. There's time later for the deeper joys I'm pointing toward, but right now, at your age, you have different goals and desires, just as the teenager has a different and appropriate purpose and view of things from her middle-aged parents. Just live out each moment of your years well, Eleanor, as passionately and mindfully as you can.

Here's a trick I use to make a decision: I imagine myself an old woman on my deathbed. I don't want ever to say at that moment, "I could have done it, and I didn't take the dare."

Take the dare, Eleanor. Take all the dares.

That's the trick to a happy old age.

Hugs,
Sophy

P.S. I came across this quote from Thich Nhat Hanh, in *Good Citizens: Creating Enlightened Society.*

When you are young person, you are like
a young creek, and you meet many rocks,
many obstacles and difficulties on your way.
You hurry to get past these obstacles and get to
the ocean. But as the creek moves down through
the fields, it becomes larger and calmer and it can
enjoy the reflection of the sky. It's wonderful.
You will arrive at the sea anyway so enjoy the journey.
Enjoy the sunshine, the sunset, the moon,
the birds, the trees, and the many beauties along
the day. Taste every moment of your daily life.

—Thich Nhat Hanh

P.P.S. Have I shown you how to see the light or aura that surrounds each living sentient thing? It's easy to see. I wrote about it in my book *The Art of Intuition*. Remind me to give you lessons when we meet next. Whenever I find myself irritated by someone, angry and annoyed (OK, I'll use those passionate words), I stop to look for the person's aura, this energy and light that we all throw out and that we live inside of—because once seen, I am reminded that she, too, this person who is so aggravating or even dangerous, is a spiritual being walking about in physical form and doing the best she can with what pathetic few tools she carries in her toolbox.

Mother-Daughters

Dear Eleanor,

You'll notice I haven't mentioned my mother, Sophy, the sister of your grandmother in these letters. The mother-daughter relationship is so close and so complex that it's hard to depict: a great mingling of love-rebellion, admiration-criticism, judgment-misunderstanding. Mine with my mother was fraught. But another reason I have not spoken of her is that she died before ever reaching "old." She was only 68 when the third bout of cancer finally felled her. I've spent the rest of my life coming to terms with her death, her courage, my anger and disappointment, and my unbounded love for the decisions that made her who she was.

The third daughter of a third daughter, she spent her life, I think, making up for the disappointment of not being a son. From this came a deep sense of inadequacy. She was never sent to college, as bright young Southern women of a certain class were not considered important enough in that time to educate. I think this hurt more than she ever admitted. She would have liked to have been a doctor, like her beloved father. Had she been a boy, of course, no expense would have been spared on her higher education, but as a woman her role from birth was marriage. Her work: to care for her household, her land (if she had any), her children, and her husband.

When I think of her, I remember her from when I was a child: how she galloped us around the kitchen, always playing, or read to us children at night before bedtime, the three of us listening quietly before the fire. I remember her restless energy, hauling the tiny tractor around the straggly grass that struggled against the acorns under the oak trees. She fed the chickens, ducks, horses, and dogs, and during the War (that's World War II) when my father was in the Pacific, she tended the one-acre victory garden that fed us. I remember once (only once) how she chopped the head off a chicken with an axe. She placed the chicken with its head on a stump and CHOP! I was probably 3 at the time, dancing from foot to foot in horrified and exhilarated fascination. Afterward she tossed the feathered body into a basket. "Is it still alive?" I trebled, watching the spasms that jerked its feet and wings. "Why is it moving, Mummy? Is it dead yet?" She explained nothing. Instead she picked up the basket and strode to the kitchen to pluck it.

Today I see how distasteful that job must have been, but I'm speaking of a time during the Depression when if you wanted to eat, you killed. In those days we didn't have markets with meters of cold cases, displaying neatly cut-up meat (removed from any recognizable animal with eyes) and packed in plastic and cellophane.

There was nothing my mother could not do: she laid and mortared the brick walkway at the back of house, created a walled brick kitchen garden with a goldfish pond. I remember her riding, too, and being proud when told she "rides like a man." She cleaned stalls, she chopped and hauled in wood for the fires, and in the evening she bathed and changed into long skirts for dinner cooked by the neighbor down the road and served on fine china with the silverware sparkling in the candlelight on a white tablecloth, my father seated at the head of the table and my mother at the foot.

And Daddy? In my childhood, the men drove off each morning to do something unimportant and unrelated to our female lives, then returned at night to shift uneasily into our matriarchal culture. My father did not lift a finger at home. No tools and handiwork for him. Indeed, the only thing I remember him doing around the Place was to take us children to chop down a straggly evergreen and drag it home on Christmas Eve and later to hang one ball on the tree before settling down with his drink to watch his chattering family trim the tree. We accepted the fact that men read or played chess while the women cared for things.

One day, when I was a young wife living in New York with tiny babies, my mother telephoned to report on the huge snowstorm that had hit. The snow came up to the window sills, she said, and the cars looked like white mushrooms, barely visible in the white expanse.

"The snow was so deep," said my mother, "that your father came to the front door to watch me pull the sledge to bring in firewood. He was that concerned."

She was truly touched.

Another time I remember sitting at the breakfast table with Daddy when he called to Mummy upstairs: "Sophy? Sophy?"

My mother clattered down the stairs in her open-heeled mules with the pink pom-poms on her toes, until she stood at the dining room door.

"Yes?"

He looked up. "Can I have more coffee?"

I was shocked. "Daddy," I said. "The coffee is right on the stove in the kitchen. Did it ever occur to you to walk out and get it?"

He looked at me, eyes wide. "No," he said. "It never did."

At the time, I was aghast. Now I look back and see how in that moment he was telling her that he loved and needed her, and she, clattering downstairs to bring him coffee, was saying it back to him.

The past is never dead. It's not even past.

—William Faulkner, *Requiem for a Nun*

My parents, both born in the first decade of the new century, were products of Edwardian reserve. Stiff upper lip. Self-reliance. Never ask for help. It was a closed and caste-ridden society, filled with formalities. My father, with experience in work and war, had learned to slough off some of this Emersonian self-reliance, but to my mother, asking for help showed weakness. I'll explain more in a moment. Child of war and the Depression, she counted her pennies. Why not? She had no other way of acquiring money— independence. Scrimp and save. A facile seamstress, she made her own clothes.

In my youth I rebelled against her conventional fears and social propriety. Today I am filled with admiration of her courage.

And then one day my father had a stroke—presenting, in the words of W. H. Auden, "thoughts of . . . death, like the distant roll of thunder at a picnic."

Soon after, she drove into town and bought three beautiful designer evening gowns. One was a skin-tight sequined black gown, another a peppermint-striped cocktail dress. I don't remember the third. She tried them on for me, twirling before my admiration.

She never wore them. When she died, they still hung in her closet in plastic covers, for right on top of Daddy's news came word of her cancer.

I learned of it afterward, in the form of an offhand comment.

"Oh, I was in the hospital."

"In the hospital! Mummy!"

"It was nothing. I didn't want to bother you children and make you worry. I'm fine." She had lopped off one breast with the disdain of a classical Amazonian determined to draw her bow. Told she would never play golf again, she taught herself to swing a golf club, even though most of the muscles on one side of her body had been removed.

Why didn't she tell me? Why take on this burden without help? I think that if she had let down her guard, received our frightened empathy, she might have wept for a thousand years. I think it was her way of protecting herself from fear.

After the breast cancer, the infection spread to her lungs. Another surgery removed a lung. She had smoked her whole life long, beginning as a girl when the doctors advised that smoking would ease her allergies and asthma.

> *. . . we must remember these people*
> *when we are safely in the future.*
> —Kate Atkinson, *Life After Life*

Lying in bed at night almost fifty years later, I can't forget the evening gowns. I want her to have worn them with her elbow-length white leather gloves to a formal dance or to the annual Baltimore Cotillion. I want her to have had the pleasure of seeing herself beautiful on Daddy's arm—he in white tie and tails, tipping his silk evening hat to us children, the crown of which folded flat with a satisfying thump. Awake and squirming with two-in-the-morning regrets, I wish that for my mother.

At the time, I promised myself not to wait: Wear the damn gown. Don't put things off. Dress up. Snatch at life. It is so short!

She died at a youthful 68, worn out by disease and the challenge of the fight.

The last thing she did was demand to leave the hospital, lugging her oxygen tank, to die in her own bed, in her beloved house, which we called the Place. A day or two after her return, she called each of us children, each of our spouses, and each of our children (her grandchildren) one by one to her bedside to say a personal goodbye.

Two days later she died. On her last night, she had somehow managed to walk down two flights to the basement to check that the pump in its Etruscan cave was still heaving and gasping (oogah, oogah), as if she were saying goodbye to the heartbeat of the house.

My sister helped her to climb back upstairs and settle again to bed. How did she do it?

The next morning she was found dead on the floor, apparently having stumbled to the window to look outside. What had she seen? One of the birds she loved? An angel taking her to the Light. I'm hurting now, typing these words. There's never enough time to express our love, enough generosity to forgive the ignorant rebellions of our youth.

She died before my father, and for the next three years we felt her presence in the house, like a scent, like a palpable energy. Twice she came back after death, showing her spirit self to me. The first time she appeared in the doorway, she was a youthful 40, in full health and happiness, loving me. I wrote about this, too, in *A Book of Angels*, and about how love breaks your heart open. But afterward, we merely felt her presence in the house, invisible, waiting for Daddy. Three years later, when Daddy died, they suddenly both left. We found ourselves saying things like, "Did you get the car for the wedding—I mean, funeral?"

We never questioned that she had waited, watching over him, until he was ready to come.

I have one more story about my mother. Showing how close we were. Before my father died, I was living in New Mexico, where I had a grant to stay at an artists' colony. One day I heard my mother's voice in my ear, telling me something about my father at nine o'clock that evening. I thought she meant to telephone him. The message repeated. Nine o'clock. I spent the day waiting to call at nine.

That evening at seven o'clock the phone rang to say that my father had just died. I was horrified. I had not yet called. It was seven o'clock in New Mexico but nine o'clock back in Baltimore. My mother had come to tell me the time of his death.

When I reached 67, I was sure that I would die that year. It seemed appropriate. How could I live longer than my mother? But that year passed, and I found myself alive, to my surprise. The next year, at 68, I bought my horse, which is itself an act of optimism, and now I've had almost twenty years of riding and loving her. Sometimes I wonder if my mother, with her love of horses, gave my mare to me.

A friend of mine told me the other day that she finds it sad that people die early, "because they don't get to see what happened to everyone." I laughed: how true. I think of my mother, who never got to see her grandchildren grow up. And then I think that of course she did. Or does. Just not as herself in the physical world. Don't I feel her all the time, even after forty years?

Grief

February 12

Dear Eleanor,

    This past weekend I went to see my dear friend Ellie, who at 91 is losing her speech. She has the beginnings of dementia. She sat on the couch in her New York City apartment, staring at the floor. I burst in, full of forced gaiety and motion, and immediately stopped. I was moving too fast. We embraced. Did she know me? I think so, although she may have lost the name, which I told her easily. "Hello, my darling. It's Sophy." She threw me her brilliant smile before moving back toward that misty zone that I associate with the shadow land of the ancient Greeks, the land that Odysseus visited, and also Aeneas, where the Shades move silently. I found myself blabbing anxiously, uneasy with silence, until I just sat calming myself, rubbing her back, and later looking at an art book with her. She was interested. That is, she looked with interest at the photographs of classical paintings. She could tell me that her elder daughter had been to visit and her other daughter was taking her to dinner that night. She could ask whether I was staying with my friends, and name them, like a burst of sunlight in a forest grove.

Yet I found myself growing more and more anxious, and finally I ran away, fleeing from the burning in my chest.

I am not proud of myself. I felt awful for not staying longer, for being unable to drink in this view of my brilliant, shining friend. I walked for long, unnecessary blocks, walking, walking, before grabbing the Metro uptown, walking to ease my distress, the loss of my friend, walking, walking, to stave off my loss and the sight of what lies ahead for me.

Ellie wrote a poignant book, *Making an Exit*, about her vital, energetic mother's voyage into Alzheimer's. It's ironic that she is drowning in that same sea.

It makes me aware of how much friendship and communication require language. Without words we are all helpless. Without words we have no thoughts, or as Maylis de Kerangal put it in *Painting Time*, "language is what allows us to see." Is friendship only the babble of exchanged ideas? I'm aware of the anxiety roiling through me, which I generously interpret as having energy, being alive. But anxiety is another word for fear.

Oh God! My friend is still inside that body but lost to me. She graduated summa cum laude from Radcliffe (Harvard, as she preferred to call it), got her Ph.D. while she and I, in our 30s, were struggling with the conflicting demands of children and career, not to mention husbands, marriage, divorce, the spiritual search, Buddhism, gurus, Christianity. She taught theater at Yale Drama School, wrote books, gave papers at conferences around the world. She was vital, electric, brilliant. We wrote long letters to each other over the years. She fell in love with a man eighteen years younger (and he with her), and after some years she managed to separate from so unsuitable a partner and take up with her present love, who loyally remains with her in these declining years.

> *. . . time heals bereavement [but] . . .*
> *Faces fade, voices dim. Seize them back . . .*
> *call their names. Do this and do not let sorrow*
> *die, for it is the sweetening of every gift.*
> —Cormac McCarthy, *The Crossing*

Now, typing this on my center island in my kitchen, I can't stop seeing her with her mind meandering into that gray zone where I cannot follow.

Yet, I'm sure she is happy. The problem lies not in her but in me, the anxiety provoked by seeing her. We were such close friends, and now here I am with nothing to say to her. What does that say about me? Pridefully, I had imagined that I was stronger, more flexible, more "spiritual" than to run away.

Afterward, the miles falling away under my feet, I walked, weeping, grateful that I can still walk, grateful that the flat, concrete sidewalks in New York make walking easy. It's been days since I've seen my friend, and I keep walking.

It's called grief.

Running from Death

Dear Eleanor,

When I was a young girl, perhaps 18 or 19, my grand-mother, then younger than I am now, suddenly turned to me. We were in her living room, I remember, and I can even now almost smell the cool, dusty scent of the old farmhouse, windows closed against the summer heat.

"I'm afraid of dying," she blurted.

Terrified, I plunged away.

I was only a kid and scared myself of death.

It sits on my heart today, my regret at having let her down. I wonder, waking in the night, what I might have said or what I would say today, from this vantage point of age. Certainly, I would not have run away.

I wish I had asked her to tell me more. I wish I'd said "Let's talk about it."

Because of course we are all afraid of our own extinguishment. Our life is the most important fact of our life, and the idea of its extinction is . . . impossible, actually, to conceive.

I wish I'd said I love you. Thank you for having been alive for me. For me, you will never die. . . .

Or we could have talked about the afterlife that she didn't believe in and that she'd given lip service to as an Episcopalian all her years. I could not have told her anything about near-death experiences, and the light and joy reported, because I learned about these only decades after her death.

What I did: I ran away.

Was it Camus who said, "As soon as you make peace with death, you will know how to live"?

Tell your friend that in his death,
a part of you dies and goes with him.
Wherever he goes, you also go.
He will not be alone.
—Jiddu Krishnamurti

When I was 24, newly married and lying in bed late at night beside my sleeping husband, the sudden comprehension hit me that I would someday die. I sat up straight in bed. The knowledge clutched my throat. Terror! Not that I didn't know about death. I knew perfectly well that everything died. But I'd never before attached the idea with such immediacy to my own self. To be extinguished? Die? How could that be? I tossed and fought for months in fruitless nighttime hours, trying to figure a way out. A plan. There MUST be a way for me not to die. I hardly slept. At night dreams woke me. In the daytime I worried the question, shaking it back and forth like a terrier with its favorite toy. Perseverating. Finally, I realized I was driving myself insane. I would be institutionalized unless I put the matter aside. It took a decision. Like Scarlett O'Hara, I'd think of it "tomorrow." Tomorrow I'd figure out what to do, tomorrow, when I knew a little more. . . .

Thoughts on his own death,
like the distant roll
of thunder at a picnic . . .
—W. H. Auden, *Marginalia*

Today, I have no fear of death. It is not only that I have glimpsed the afterlife but also that so many spirits, complete with character and personality, have come to me while working as a medium that I am convinced we do not vanish utterly. Matter and energy cannot be extinguished. Indeed, my comfort runs deeper than that. Somehow, over the years, I've befriended death. Without death, I would not be as content as now, right this minute, aware that everything is transient, impermanent, including me. It makes every moment precious, Eleanor. For never again will this moment return. (Oops, gone!) Perhaps this is another gift of old age, although wise gurus have been teaching it for millennia: this moment. Now. Be here now. More important, be aware of being here NOW.

On the other hand, I am aghast at the irony that it is our very strengths that seem to be taken in old age. In the case of my father, who loved above all to discuss and dispute in intellectual argumentation (if possible before the Supreme Court), it was speech that was removed in a series of strokes and tiny electrical burnouts, like a house slowly going dark. And for my brilliant friend, Ellie, with her summa cum laude at Harvard, it's the similar ability in dementia to form articulate thoughts. For one athlete I know, it is physical activity that goes, as he has lost balance and spinal security.

I boast I'm not afraid of dying, but what I am afraid of, Eleanor, is the pain that seems always to accompany the passage into death. Perhaps we would never leave our bodies without the pain; I don't know. But what we do to humans who are dying is barbaric: I want a vet at my bedside when I die.

I have had the privilege to "put down" (as we call it) several dear dogs and my beloved cat and even one horse, and it is a beautiful, gentle, tender way to go. When we have the ability to help our darling to go quietly to sleep as we hold and pet him, talking soothingly of our love and thanks, and when, once sleep has fallen, we allow the vet to give the final injection that sends our beloved painlessly across the River Styx while we weep and shudder with love and letting go, and afterward when we hold the still-warm body with further kisses and goodbyes—then we know the death was good.

I'll tell two stories. This is how I know I'm not afraid of death itself.

---

*You get old and you realize
there are no answers, just stories.*
—Garrison Keillor, *Pontoon: A Novel of Lake Wobegon*

Not long ago I participated with two friends in a kind of spiritual or healing session using bowls and gongs. One gong was as tall as I, with a voice to shake the gods. Lying on a mat on the floor, feeling the deep reverberating booming in the bones of my body, I found myself going deep inside, down, down—until suddenly I found myself, as if outside my body and watching thoughts slide and slither through my mind, and it occurred to me, lazily, that that's all I am: my thoughts, coupled perhaps with my sense of self-consciousness or of "me." Turning the axiom of Descartes around, I'd say, "I am because I think." Lying, eyes closed, I understood that truly the world would miss nothing when my thoughts slip into oblivion with death. They are nothing that everyone else doesn't think . . . or hasn't thought since the world began. It will be OK for me to go.

"So you were divorced from your thinking?" my friend asked curiously when I described it later. But no, I was still conscious of myself watching myself. Therefore, I still contained "thought." Or entertained thoughts. I still had thoughts. What I felt was that dying won't be bad—as if I have only to let go of one more onion layer of self-importance.

I have spent a lifetime pondering: Who am I? Why am I here? And what am I supposed to be doing? And what about death or letting go? Will it be only out of intolerable pain that I will be willing to step into the Void?

Of course this is nonsense. Life is more than merely thoughts. My friend hidden in her dementia is still herself, moving in worlds she cannot describe or perhaps remember or perhaps that I cannot hear. So, likewise, is my mute autistic nephew who is vibrantly alive and communicating without the help of words.

"Language and thought," says Ev Fedorenko, an MIT neuroscientist, "are separate in an adult brain."

That's amazing! Thinking thoughts and decoding words mobilize different pathways in the brain, but both thinking and decoding represent only one small part of who we are. More than thinking will go with us when we pass over. But I have no idea what it is—an essence, perhaps?

Animals talk, sometimes vocalizing physically like birds or dogs or whales, and sometimes by telepathy, sending wordless images of the stories or pain or triumphs that they want to tell. This silent imagery is what I am "watching" when giving a psychic reading and struggling to translate it into words. This is what animal communicators hear when listening to a cat or horse. What part of our brains picks up these soundless thoughts?

But I was talking about how I'm unafraid of death. A while ago I was in Washington, D.C., happily in bed asleep, when I was awakened by a tearing, searing pain in my chest. I lay in bed, deliberating. "It's not a surface pain," I reflected. "It feels like a muscle deep in my chest. My heart?" If it was a heart attack, I should call 911. But lying there, I knew that if I got out of bed to find my phone downstairs, I'd fall on the floor, unable to move. That's how exhausted I felt, so tired I might as well stay in bed. Next, I considered: It's okay, my affairs are all in order. If I'm alive in the morning and still have this pain, I'll go to the ER.

Eventually, despite the pain, I fell back to sleep.

In the morning the tearing sensation, like ripping a piece of paper in two, still violently hurt. I took myself to the ER, where, of course, the moment I touched the hospital door, the pain stopped. I spent the entire day at Sibley Hospital being given tests. It turns out there is nothing wrong with my heart, but I do have a blood clot in one leg that could travel to my lungs and kill me. For weeks I had been ignoring my swollen leg and ankle and the burst blood vessels at my knee.

The funny thing about facing imminent death is that it really snaps everything else into perspective.

—James Patterson, *The Angel Experience*

I burst out laughing. I could just imagine my angels and spirit guides working overtime to produce yet another miracle (I've had so many!)—this time a fake heart attack to force me to the ER! (Later I learned that heart pain is one sign of a blood clot, no angels needed.) I tell you this, Eleanor, because it reinforces my impression that I'm not afraid to die. It's not something I'm hurrying toward but evidently nothing I'm frightened of either—not even enough to climb out of bed.

On the other hand, death—I keep saying this—is what makes this period of my life so precious, this heightened awareness of how little time is left. I have, how many—ten years left? Twelve? I don't have time to waste on anger and resentment anymore, nor on self-pity or pessimism or despair. I know a woman who counts her days: she has only four thousand more days to live, she says, if she lives to 95.

Of course it's not only the aged and elderly but young folk, too, who understand and make use of death breathing at our back.

My sister-in-law, Sue, and her husband fought for decades like cats tied in a sack together—until Sam got cancer. He was given three to six months to live. He lived another six years, and in that time, they fell in love all over again. It was beautiful to watch. But what felt different to them? Nothing but the sudden realization, principally on Sue's part, that life is fragile, transient, impermanent. She fell head over heels in love with her husband all over again—and what a waste those years of bickering.

So, yes! I say to life yes, and yes, and yes to all the misery that turns into joy, and all the goodness shining in the midst of fear: the goodness of people, just ordinary little moments like the grocery clerk today who called me "honey," smiling with her snaggletooth and blue braces as she handed me my receipt.

Imagine, I get to have the experience of that!

Instead of possibilities, I have realities in my past, not only the reality of work done and of love loved, but of suffering suffered. These are things of which I am most proud, though these are things which cannot inspire envy.

—Victor E. Frankl, *Man's Search for Meaning*

Recently, two people on the same day announced to me that they wanted to live to 150 and saw no reason why it was not feasible. I was aghast. "Why in the world would anyone want to live that long?" But holding my tongue, I asked simply, "Why?"

"I'm just not ready to die."

I didn't point out that hardly anyone is ready to die, but that living past, say, 105 brings its own distress. All your friends have died before you, and possibly your children. You are alone and perhaps hardly able to lift your fork without spilling down your beard, so that someone else must feed you as well as change your diapers. You nap like a newborn, and, if you are lucky, you may still have your mind intact and speech. But what good is that if your back hurts? Your knees don't work. You have no balance. You can't stand up straight anymore but crouch forward like an Allen key. You lose names or confuse generations, thinking your great-nephew is your brother, or your daughter a stranger.

The ones who want to live that long are dreaming of having it together with the energy of health and youth.

There's a common saying, "Old age is not for sissies."

It's one more of those misleading aphorisms that we learn as children, such as "Opportunity comes but once." (Nonsense! Life is not so chary: opportunities come again and again, blessings poured upon us boundlessly, if only we are alert enough to see. It's up to us to grab at them.)

As for old age, dummy, *life* is not for sissies!

Every year delivers insuperable challenges. My God, what's harder than being a baby struggling to pull herself up on her feet—and falling, plunk, each time? Or being a teenager navigating life? It's how we meet the challenges that determines who we are.

Waiting for the Doorbell

Even when I'm making a risotto,
Even when cleaning my fingernails
Or admiring the gaudy sunset spread
Across a vulgar sky,
I have one ear cocked for the doorbell.
Now?
Or maybe now?
I think while the clock tick-
Tocks its time.
Because he will come soon, I know.
(But why do I say "he"?)

Wrapped in a black cloak,
Designer made, no doubt,
And maybe a black beret perched on her
Dyed-blonde hair, the
Flash of eyes—
She'll have a huge warm smile
(Skin like a 10-year old,
All bloom and silken smooth).
Are you ready? She'll sing—

"Ready? NO!
I have to empty the dishwasher still
And write my granddaughter—so much I haven't had time
To tell her, and cuddle the cat,
No. Wait. Come in.
Have a cup
Of tea. I have so much to do."

Come on, you'll like it.
Her lilting laughter
Light as air. She'll reach out one perfect
Manicured hand, touch me, and
She is seduction. Eros. Aphrodite. I leave
The door open in my hurry, and the dishes
Unwashed and the wet ink blotting
On the page, dirty clothes in the
Hamper, the bed unmade, and nothing finished
Because all I want is to follow her.

Meanwhile, how sweet to make risotto, adding cheese,
The curve of a blanket fold, the plunk
Of flowers in a vase,
The flicker of a swallow's tail,
The gray squirrel swarming up the tree,
The wind tossing down the grass like long-haired girls.

It's enough to make you wish
The doorbell would never ring—

But no, such things are only dear because I know
That soon, too soon,
I'll hear her at the door, the urgent peal, her shining face—
"Like your cloak," I'll say, rejoicing
As we move
Together
Hand in hand.

—Sophy Burnham

Too Old!

March 2

Oh, Eleanor, I've been talking about how interesting this stage of life is as an old woman. On the other hand, I look at our political leaders and I'm disgusted. They are TOO OLD! What's the matter with them? Don't they know when to leave the stage? Leave the work to the 40- and 60-year-olds, full of ignorance and energy. This is the oldest Congress in history. As I write this: Mitch McConnell is 80, Biden turning 80, Trump 77. In Congress we have Diane Feinstein (D) 90, Chuck Grassley (R) 88, Richard Shelby (R) 86, Patrick Leahy (D) 80, Jim Inhofe (R) 86, and another twenty-one members who are in their late or mid-70s. Dear God! These are the people governing us, and YES! They are my age, and YES, they are too old. One has dementia, another's mind is freezing up, another suffered a stroke that makes his speaking difficult.

They should withdraw into the role of "advisors" or wise elders, not cling to power, as if they have no identity beyond the title of their job.

What I'm saying is that there is a time to work like a donkey, back laden with the sticks and fagots for the fire, and a time for standing on the sidelines.

"Leave the dance," my mother always counseled, "while you're still having a good time."

Today the local paper reported on the Veteran of the Year, a World War II servicewoman, now 101. (At least she is not running for office.) It makes me mad just to think of our aged members of Congress refusing to let go. Or the courts. Look at Ruth Bader G., who was too scared to step down. Look at the havoc her ego spread.

I won't say anything about Biden running for office for another four years, the decision of a man surely losing his grip, or the Other likewise running. What is the matter with people (and I mean the voters, the "selectors")?

Isn't one part of wisdom simply acceptance? Accepting reality, by which I mean not grudging resignation but passionate, joyful, open-armed embrace of the next adventure? I suppose the politicians would say they actually do accept their reality—which is that no one else can do their job! And thus they will stay in harness until they fall down dead.

Today I woke up to gray misty skies and rain, clouds boiling inside me as well as out. I went to the stable to watch a 10-year-old girl, Sabine, ride my horse in a lesson (nice hands, good balance). Being a WASP to whom exercise is the answer to everything, I cleaned out Spring's stall just for the pleasure of physical labor, lifting manure on the fork, heaving it into the wheelbarrow, and then wheeling the heavy barrow to the manure pile.

But man, proud man,
Drest in a little brief authority,
Most ignorant of what he's most assured
His glassy essence, like an angry ape
Plays such fantastic tricks before high heaven
As makes the angels weep[.]
—William Shakespeare, *Measure for Measure*

I still felt vile.

I'm supposed to be doing. And do little.

I tell myself I'm lazy. I'm no good.

Today's *New York Times* has an article about Frederick Wiseman, a documentary filmmaker who just finished a new film at age 91, having produced one a year for fifty-five years. Now, for the first time in fifty-five years, he's not working on a new project.

"In addition to being scared," he is quoted as saying, "I'm bored."

Maybe that's me today: maybe I'm bored.

I'm ashamed of myself. Imagine being bored!
What a waste.

Maybe that's why the politicians don't quit. They're
afraid of feeling useless. Or bored. And here's another interesting thing: it doesn't matter how much you have done in
life, how many accolades and awards you have received,
how many compliments and kudos—in the end they are all
unimportant. I remember my beloved boss Roger Stevens,
the Broadway producer, then in his mid-80s, remarking as
he received another award, "That's what they do when they
think you're finished: give another award."

He had received dozens by then, including knighthood
by the Queen of England. It was living that interested him.

Roger never attended college. The Depression forced him
to go to work in a Ford assembly line in order to send his
siblings through school and college. He made a fortune in New
York real estate, one of his deals being to buy and then sell
the Empire State Building. Enormously wealthy, self-taught,
highly educated, vibrant, charismatic, he became, out of love of
theater, a Broadway producer, and we owe to Roger more than
a hundred plays and musicals supporting works by people
like Tennessee Williams, Tony Kushner, Tom Stoppard. By
the time I came along (as director of his pet project, the Fund

for New American Plays), he was in his 80s, retired, restless, engaged, and still energetic as he worked from his enormous office in the John F. Kennedy Center for the Performing Arts, which as chairman he had raised the money to construct.

I was struck by how he funded his projects—not with his own money. He'd shout to his secretary, "Get me Max on the phone," for he'd had a stroke and his fingers could no longer dial the tiny numbers on a phone.

"Max!" he'd shout joyfully. "I've got a great idea for you. Put money into *Les Misérables*." And then came the kicker, the one that poured money into his hands: "It will be fun!"

Oh, I learned a lot from Roger. I was in my 50s at the time and half in love with him. He was captivating. After one meeting, for example, I said I'd type up notes.

"No, no." He stopped me. "Put nothing in writing."

"How can you prove what was agreed, in case there's a dispute?"

He tapped his temple, eyes twinkling. "I have it all up here."

I typed the notes anyway, just in case. They were never needed.

As for the idea of politicians afraid of feeling useless or being bored, my mother used to tell me there is no excuse for being bored.

"If you are bored," she'd say, "you aren't paying attention. No one is boring. You're not paying attention. Listen harder. Wake up."

The fact is there's nothing boring about this period of octogenarian old age.

And so I wonder, remembering Roger and his active curiosity, why I feel so passionate about the aged politicians making decisions for us. Is it my own ageism? Or is it practicality, knowing from experience what it's like at 85, 86, and how often I see the elderly curl lazily into their comfort? I know I'm slowing down. I sometimes take a nap in the afternoon.

I'm back to mindfulness. This breath. And this next one. And this, until I see—really see—the crows flying overhead, until I become the winter tree with its twisted arms and burls, the cancerous growths on its beautiful bark, until I am—how did I miss it?—the tree, the robin strutting on the frozen grass. We are interdependent. Bored, delighted, sad, glad, active, restless, jealous, worried. So what? They are only feelings, throwing themselves onto the beach like ocean waves and being sucked out, each emotion replaced by another wave. As we are replaced. How right, how rich, how just, how inexorable, how inevitable is life.

This breath.

What We Talk About When We Talk in Old Age

March 29

Dear Eleanor,

Do you remember my writing about the woman with dementia whom I walked with one day in my walking group? How angry I was at being classified as "old"? We've become friends. I play chess with her. She can't always remember how the pieces move, and she confuses the king and queen, but she is so willing ("Is this a good move?" she asks in hesitant appeal) that who could be annoyed? She's charming. She doesn't know she has dementia. It's nice for me to find a path to win, even if I give her a queen and bishop handicap. Moreover, playing chess with her gives her daughter a few free hours to have tea with a friend or to catch up on paperwork.

How curious life is. Who would have guessed that I'd become friends with a woman in dementia.

I wish I'd done as well with my dear friend in New York.

Today I went to play chess with her. Her sharp eyes glare like a peregrine falcon, suspicious, cautious. I can see that she was once formidable. She is on the alert, knowing something's wrong even if she's not sure what.

After a few games, we paused. "I want to ask you something," I began, hoping to interview her. "I've been thinking lately about being old. I'm old. What do you think about being old?"

"I don't think about it," she said, and then rearing in fearless attack: "I think about my apartment in New York. I want to live there. I don't want to be here, but my daughter—two daughters—insist. They say I can't live alone. I'm 89 years old, and I've lived in New York most of my life. I taught right up until last spring."

"What did you teach?"

"Art history. I taught at New York University for thirty years."

"Oh, tenured?"

"No."

She went on to explain, eyes flashing with anger, that they let her go last spring. "I'm 89. I taught for thirty years. I could have kept on."

"Ageism?"

"Exactly."

"Are you angry?" Her whole body was tensed, shoulders tight.

"Yes, I'm angry. Wouldn't you be?"

"Going back to being old, do you notice any difference?"

"No. I don't think about my age. I'm not any different. I don't feel different. I feel 40 or 50." She laughed and proudly proclaimed. "I walk. I walk a lot."

Abashed, I recognize in her my own pride and denial of aging. I laughed with her that I don't feel my age either. I, too, feel only about 50 inside, but I notice changes.

"Like what?" Her questions are shotgun explosions. Aggressive. Are they hiding curiosity or a secret need for knowledge?

"I don't run up the stairs anymore, ride my bike, ski."

"Oh, well." We laughed.

"And what about dying? What do you think about dying?"

"I don't want to do it," she snapped, quick as a whip. We talked more about death and the possibility of afterlife, but she had set her mind years earlier on these matters and wasn't about to change it. When you aren't sure of your mind, you keep it on a tight leash. "When you die, you're gone," she proclaimed with the certainty of a Ph.D. who taught for thirty years.

Then we turned back to the chess game. "Is this a good move?"

I was struck by how modest she had become, how completely she lives in the present. Is that the gift of dementia? To live entirely in Right This Minute, Now?

You know what we talk about, the friends my age? We talk about politics, climate change, corruption, the Supreme Court. Many of my younger friends in their 50s and 60s and 70s have almost no interest in politics. They talk about each other, and I have the impression they don't even follow the news with more than desultory interest, but when I get together once a week with my coven of witches, all of us over 80, we talk about women who are raped by lawless gangs in Haiti, or in Iraq, Afghanistan, Ukraine, Congo— wherever there is war. What is it about men in war that they have to plunge their @#*%$^ into some girl's soft parts? What psychological wound is trying to be healed?

We talk about the politicians in one state, who rejected federal (free) health care or free food for hungry children— because they don't want to make people "dependent," and anyway, there's a child obesity problem in America.

How can they sleep at night?

We talk of the rise of neo-Nazis, those of us who remember what happened in Germany under Hitler. Is anti-Semitism on the rise? We talk about guns and violence and the ethics of a Second Amendment interpreted without regard to its first thirteen words. In the U.S., 7,000 soldiers were killed in the 18 years of war in Iraq and Afghanistan, but in that same period 18,000 women were killed in the United States. That's close to three women killed every day (!) and most by current or former intimate partners. Since the end of *Roe v. Wade*, 14,000 women have died in childbirth. We think it will get worse. (Do you remember our infant mortality rate? It's 49.5 out of every 100,000 for African American babies, 22 per 100,000 for white babies, while Norway has a zero infant mortality rate.)

Kofi Annan, former U.N. secretary-general, says, "There is no policy more effective in promoting development, health and education than the empowerment of women and girls. And . . . no policy is more important in preventing conflict or in achieving reconciliation after a conflict has ended."

Women may be the one social group
that grows more radical with age.
—Gloria Steinem, *Outrageous Acts and Everyday Rebellions*

Years ago, I marched down Fifth Avenue with the Women's Movement. It was thrilling. I was one of the furious media women who "occupied" the offices of the *Ladies' Home Journal,* demanding that some of the editors of this woman's magazine should be women! (They were all men.) And demanding equal pay for women. I was in a consciousness-raising group with Susan Brownmiller, whose book *Against Our Will: Men, Women and Rape* profoundly moved me. A few years earlier, living in Washington in 1963, I had slipped down to the March on Washington, where Martin Luther King Jr. gave his speech. There were so many people at the Reflecting Pool that I could hear nothing, but standing in that sea of Black faces, I knew I was witnessing something special. I didn't know enough to call it history.

Today, we elders talk about "character," a word we don't hear much anymore. We witches talk about sending energy and casting spells against those in Congress who threaten to bring down the government they are supposed to serve, as if "the government" were some outside doomsday entity and not "We the People." Isn't that treason, we ask in confusion? How can you NOT raise the debt ceiling? How can one small individual hold up three hundred military appointments?

My younger friends don't show any interest in such things.

It might explain why it's the ancient gray-hairs who work at the voting and polling booths. And vote.

One octogenarian friend of mine, a physicist, is exploring a single question: what is life? We know about carbon atoms and stardust gases; we know about single-celled organisms arising billions of years ago. But how? Or why? And while on the topic, what of the miraculous translucence of water that allows more of the green wavelengths to pass through water than any other color on the light spectrum? Without green, the photosynthesizing algae would not have grown, nor the one-celled creations that developed into multiple-celled forms. What are the chances of translucent water allowing mostly the single color green to pass unhindered?

We talk, my aged friends and I, about the arts and our own efforts to produce our art, and also about prayer and the spiritual life, of the holiness of trees and earth, how everything is sacred and everything is calling us: grasses, trees, earthworms, ants, spiders, flowers, rocks, and stones. If we had ears sensitive enough, we could probably hear them sing, including the waves that batter themselves against the boulders on the beach.

We talk of beauty.

We talk of beauty everywhere.

Rarely do we talk about the past.

Remember that I told you, Eleanor, how sorry I am that I never asked Gaga or my aunts more about their early lives? I remember asking Aunt Kate what it was like when she was growing up. I wanted to hear how, in the years before the First World War, she and her sisters, dressed in their little sailor blouses, would walk with their mother down 16th Street to the White House to call on the president's wife, poor thing, who had no social life. They would leave my grandmother's calling card on a silver platter in the hall, and in a few days the First Lady would invite her with her husband, the Doctor, to the White House or to a private dinner at Decatur Place. The custom stopped in the early '20s. I wanted to hear about taking a train across the country at the end of WWI to spend the summer at a Montana dude ranch, or how she had lived in Majorca for a few years before coming home to marry Uncle Dick. What was she doing there? Did she fall in love?

In spite of illness, in spite even of the archenemy sorrow, one can remain alive long past the usual date of disintegration if one is unafraid of change, insatiable in intellectual curiosity, interested in big things, and happy in small ways.
—Edith Wharton, *A Backwards Glance*

At 94, Aunt Kate had no interest in the past. She was too involved with Spanish lessons, nature shows on TV, politics, gossip with friends.

I refuse to be intimidated by reality anymore.

—Lily Tomlin

Now I understand: the present is fascinating.

These days I want to talk about my grandchildren, each one different and fully formed: Adelaide, who all her life has wanted to be an actress; Beatrice, the mathematician and scientist; Georgia, with her artistic abilities and her quiet observing of whatever is going on. Oh, she's filled with surprises, that one! And all of them alive with the beauty and energy of youth. But none has taught me so much as my valiant Michael. I know nothing about being a grandmother, but let anyone touch one hair of their heads and I'll kill to defend them. (So much for absence of passion.)

Once I took my grandson on a picnic to a lovely pond nearby. As we ate our sandwiches, curious, I asked, "You're 9 years old. You're pretty big. What advice and counsel would you give to your littler self, when you were, let's say, 5?"

"Oh, that's a big question," he said, chewing thoughtfully. "I'd have to think about that." After a few minutes, he decided:

"First, be yourself. Don't think you have to be or do what someone else thinks just because they want you to be that way. Be your Self.

"Second, if you see a bully in the playground pushing around a littler kid, go up to him and say, 'Why are you doing this? You don't have to be mean to littler kids.'"

These two answers started such a discussion that we never got around to number three. But I was struck by his claim for authenticity. Is anything more important than this search for authentic identity?

Still, I'm not the only grandmother coming to terms with changes that shake the very foundations of our ingrained values. The world is changing so fast: technology, geography, weather, communications, customs, ethics, values, beliefs. Everything seems up for grabs. Even a TikTok now passes as a thank-you note for the latest generation, if you're lucky enough to get one.

"Nonsense!" my mother would have cried. "I won't hear of such a thing. Write a letter!"

Good luck with that, Mummy. It's we old hags who need most nimbly to adjust. Yet still we're called to instruct them: write or phone your thank-you. How else does the giver know her gift was received? How else can the energy of love flow back and forth between you, circulating and increasing?

What is feminine? Masculine? What is gender, sex? Are we all on a sliding musical scale of sexuality and sensuality, capable of everything? I know one boy who continues to dress partly as a girl. Or with his own creative fashion sense.

> *In all affairs it's a healthy thing now and then*
> *to hang a question mark on the things*
> *you have long taken for granted.*
> —Bertrand Russell (1872–1970)

"Clothing is simply a cultural decision," he concludes with a decisiveness that leaves me blinking. "The way you dress— fashions change all the time."

He's right, of course. Only a few hundred years ago dukes and kings dressed in peacock silks and lace and brilliant colors, in high-heeled shoes and wigs and heavy makeup.

"Do the boys at your middle school also wear skirts— besides kilts?" I asked.

"Some. In high school, too."

I couldn't believe it. I asked his older sister. "Is it true that the boys in your high school wear skirts?"

"Sure," she smiled. "I think it's sexy."

Oh, wow.

In my short time on earth, I feel as if I've lived three different lives, each swept away by the breakers of Time. There was my landed gentry childhood of the 1930s, '40s, and '50s, complete with horses and dogs, cockfighting and hard-drinking, hard-driving, cigarette-smoking adults, a time of debutante dances and little dress hats with veils, white gloves, and "manners," coupled with decisive, unquestioned beliefs and certitudes that covered anxiety and addictions. My second life contained marriage and children and struggling for a career in New York City and Washington, D.C., a period of protest and riots, Civil Rights, women's liberation, four (or more) political assassinations, the Vietnam War, a time of demonstrations and calls for freedom, of Kent State killings, police violence, and cities set aflame. This period includes the years of divorce and the urgency of my spiritual search in my 30s and 40s and a constant questioning and freeing from restraints.

*Perhaps this was part of growing older,
to undergo hideous alterations in the deepest
certainties, in love, in lovers, finally in one's self.*
—Elizabeth Harrower, *In Certain Circles*

I've seen such wonderous things in my life: I have driven a subway car, sailed an ocean liner past the Nantucket lighthouse, flown a plane in Spain (the passengers crouched terrified in their seat belts as I flirted with the pilot). I have traveled in twenty-four countries, searched for enlightenment, talked with the Dalai Lama. . . .

Today I stand in the third stage of old age. It is a time of simplifying, shedding of pretensions, searching always for the grit of truth. It's a time when the world once again is hunching its back, lurching, heaving with change, and I am required yet again to hold on tight, let go of outdated preconceptions, adjust my grip, and whoop with delight at the latest wild, free bronco ride.

Hope is definitely not the same thing as optimism. It is not the conviction that something will turn out well, but the certainty that something makes sense, regardless of how it turns out.
—Václav Havel, *Disturbing the Peace*

Looking back, I have the impression that it all makes sense. I can't quite explain it, but under every triumph, every difficulty, under all the tears and sorrow and disappointments I have lived through, under all the seeds of anguish and unhappiness, can be heard a gushing river of goodness. Good is constantly blooming from disappointment, love from bitterness. I'm back to the beginning, back to the psalms. "The Lord is my shepherd, I shall not [remain in] want. Yea, though I walk through the valley of the shadow of death, I shall fear no evil. . . ."

It's all been so good. And underneath of everything lies Love. It is an unfathomable, deep ringing bell.

What We Do When We Are Very Old

April 10

Dearest Eleanor,

Your friend Sara came to visit, as you had suggested to her. We had tea together before the gas fireplace and talked politely on superficial topics the way semi-strangers do, until it was time for her to go. Have you noticed how so often we bring up the most important topic only when standing at the door to leave? I call it the Front Door Syndrome. Leaving, saying last goodbyes, Sara suddenly blurted out her anger at her mother, whom she was driving to visit, and her anguish about her childhood.

We came back inside.

We sat on the two high stools in the kitchen, our elbows on the center island, while she stared out the porch door, unseeing or, rather, lost in her own inner landscape. I knew her story. Years earlier, I had watched her father fall in love with her mother at the family swimming pool. I'd heard of her father's death and how her mother remarried a man who had helped her through her grief, and even later I heard about the new husband's preying on her little daughters. She put the man in jail. Brave woman! I had heard about all that through the grapevine, and here was her daughter, your friend, sitting in my kitchen, pouring out her fury at her mother.

I listened.

That's what I do now.

Sara was in one of those states where she needed someone to pour her pain onto, someone safe, someone whom she might never meet again.

She confessed that she had never forgiven her mother, and anyway, she didn't know how to forgive her not only for what had happened to herself and to her sisters but for not "being there," as she put it, for not having talked intimately when she had needed it, and now for sliding toward dementia. I listened, nodding.

I knew her mother only slightly. I'd always found her practical, pragmatic, down-to-earth. I rather dismissed her as unimaginative and certainly (though this may have been ignorance on my part) uninterested in the interior life and spiritual search that means so much to you, Eleanor, and me. These are the doers who take out the garbage and call the repairmen, and God knows we're lucky to have people like that to handle mundane things while we daydreaming searchers go on fruitless explorations.

I offered Sara the Buddhist Metta prayer.

Christ tells us to forgive our brother and even our worst enemies, but he never told us how. The Buddha, on the other hand, gives exact directions, step by step. I think we talked a little about how to lift the veil of pain, how to forgive herself first and then her mother for disappointing her by basically being who she is instead of who Sara wishes that she were.

Sara described her mother's present failing condition and her own inability to talk with her as she wished, in part because of geographic distance, in part because of WASP reserve, and now the addition of early dementia.

"It's grief," I murmured at a certain moment, suddenly understanding what lay underneath her rage. "You're grieving."

I don't know whether she heard.

That's what we do in old age. We listen deeply.

Then it was time for her to leave. I watched from the door as she set out on her long drive Midwest to meet her mother.

Today, Eleanor, I got an email from Sara. She thanked me for tea and said she'd had the best visit with her mother and her mother's boyfriend that she'd ever had.

You see? There's the goodness underneath it all.

The love.

We just have to sometimes dig for it.

This is the thing about old age. I'm not the only one to find myself inadvertently guiding others, often strangers, but these days it seems to be done mostly one-on-one, as with Sara, and so quietly that I hardly know anything has happened. Sometimes the guidance is obvious, through my psychic or intuitive readings, or when I'm mentoring a younger woman (and everyone is younger) as I do in AA (they call it "sponsoring"), or through the program I instituted in the women's jail. But sometimes it's simply in casual conversation, like the woman, Linda, who came up to me a few weeks ago, to say: "Oh, I'm so glad to see you. I feel so lost today."

Often all I'm doing is listening, nodding, murmuring hmm-mm, and acting as a channel, as it were, for her to come to some recognition or realization as she talks.

I have no single wisdom to impart. If I offer guidance, it is suitable to that one person in that particular moment or situation. To another, the very opposite might apply. To one I offer Acceptance, to another Courageous Confrontation; to one I say examine and admit your part and to another speak out forcibly, demanding respect. What I'm saying is that there is no universal wisdom, unless it be that time heals most wounds and forgiving yourself and then everyone else is always appropriate if the goal is happiness.

Three grand essentials to happiness in this life are something to do, something to love, and something to hope for.

—Joseph Addison

We hear so often how our culture dismisses or disrespects older people.

It is not my experience.

I am touched by how kind people are. The other day in New York, more than one man rushed to help me with my suitcase on the subway, or to hold a door, or to give directions. "You take the cab," said one woman, laughing. "I'll catch the next one." And at one fast-food health store, a customer leapt forward to suggest that one dish is especially delicious. Little acts of kindness everywhere.

The nourishment of the body is food, while the nourishment of the soul is feeding others.

—Ali ibn Abi Talib, seventh-century Islamic caliph

163

I don't know if any of this is helpful, Eleanor. What I'm trying to say, over and over, is—don't be afraid of getting old. You can't imagine the profound understanding, the happiness, the deep, ringing joy it brings. Just hope you live long enough to experience it!

With all my love,
Sophy

Shedding, Stripping, Shifting

May 4

Dearest Eleanor,

It has been so long since I have written that much
water has flowed by in the rivers of Time. Springtime has
hit, and the garden is alive with pink and purple and white.
The peonies are glorious. (I'm so pleased: I've always
wanted peonies.) And so are the weeds. Plentiful rain
has made things thrive. I'm sleeping outside now on my
screened porch, as everyone did when we were children.
Am I trying to reconstruct my childhood, I wonder idly,
and then give in to the pleasure of the nighttime insects
screaming, of the wind in the trees, and of the special
delight of waking in the glow of first light and watching
the day swell pridefully outside? I am so deaf now that I
cannot hear the birds without my hearing aids, and even
then, I sometimes cannot hear the highest fluted calls.
No matter. I have a Cornell University app on my phone,
called Merlin, that records which birds are singing near
me and plays them right into my hearing aids: robins,
cardinals, wrens.

I think how fifty years ago I would never have heard a songbird again.

Now the bad news, Eleanor. I will not be in France with the others for the family wedding this summer. Last April a blood clot was discovered, a deep vein thrombosis. My leg is swollen, elephantine. My foot is the size of a pigeon, while broken blood vessels pour deep purple at my knee. Nonetheless the clot (tamed now on medication) is not a hindrance, not important, except that I'm not allowed on a plane. I'm sorry about that and, in a curious way, relieved. I have so much to do.

Still, I am glad the children (I call them children, my over-50 adults) will stay some of the time with you, and in September, when my blood clot has been absorbed, I will come over and we will have lunch again, before I head off with my chess group to play tournaments in Paris and London. September will mark one full year since you asked me about getting older, setting me off on this journey of exploration: what's it like to be old?

One of the most interesting results is that over these months, telling out loud how much I hate aging, everything has changed. I don't care about it at all. I'm no longer fearful or ashamed. In fact, I mostly don't think about it. I'm slowing down. So what?

It seems impossible that only eight or nine months ago I was jumping my horse over the outdoor course, still riding like a kid. Already I find it harder to heave the heavy dressage saddle up over my head and onto my horse's back. I ride, but I no longer gallop flat out, forehead low on her neck, my fingers entwined in her mane. Even so, today I rode quietly out into the fields and woods, happy just to be on my horse's back.

Recently, I moved Spring to a new barn, where they teach "Liberty." Now with the help of the incomparable teacher Meg, I get to play with my horse in new ways as she learns various tricks without a halter or lead. I'm so proud of her! In only a few lessons, she has learned to stand on a tiny platform with all four feet, balancing herself precariously with tail and neck. She has learned to kick a ball, to kneel, and also to bow, which is the first step to lying down on command.

To my delight we are also teaching her the Spanish walk, in which she lifts each front leg and throws it far ahead of her. She loves this one. Years ago, when she was just a baby, I tried to teach her this beautiful step, but without a teacher I could take her only so far. Now, with the help of Meg, I am learning to give directions on her back with my hands and seat.

Meg is a true horse whisperer. She buys wild mustangs, and in only a few weeks she has so tamed and steadied them that she can sell them as riding horses.

Meanwhile I still ride together "out" with one friend, our two mares, themselves companions, walking side by side in comfortable communication, while we riders discuss our problems, confess, advise, listen, make plans. What a magical world. What a wonderful way to live.

So those are my days, and you can see how very different they are from even a year ago, when I would ride alone, jumping logs in the woods or cantering down dirt roads. I don't do that anymore.

I don't feel I'm giving anything up. Rather, the desire has dropped away, as if it were a coat I no longer need. On the other hand, simply to be in the forgiving presence of horse energy, to groom my horse or lean on her shoulder companionably while she grazes, or else to learn the commands I need to perform Liberty—all this keeps me balanced, sane.

I wish I could come with the others for the wedding, but I will see you in September. Promise.

I look forward to lunch at that lovely little side-street café and sharing our thoughts, to seeing how you are—now that you have passed the dreaded marker of the number 60.

With love and anticipation,
Sophy

Loneliness

Dear Eleanor,

Not long ago I came across an article in the *Harvard Business Review* by Vice Admiral Vivek H. Murthy, former surgeon general, about how we live in the most technologically connected age in the history of civilization, yet rates of loneliness have doubled since the 1980s, when we suffered no computers or social media, when no one looked all day at a handheld screen. (He's written a book about this plague of our times.) Over 40 percent of adults in America today, he says, report feeling lonely, and the real number may be higher.

He's not talking necessarily about the elderly or old. He means young men and women in college, or else just starting their careers, or else suffering the middle-age rebooting of their ambitions, or else mothers with young children and husbands, juggling both careers and family and no time for themselves.

Who was it who once joked with me that if you want to be lonely, get married?

It is a truth generally accepted that old age leads to lone-liness or, put another way, that you will be lonelier in old age than ever in your life before. This is not my experience, but my heart goes out to those in nursing homes, forgotten or abandoned, unvisited by family or friends. It is true that it may be harder to make friends as you get older, but no one in my little circle of interviews expressed any sense of loneliness or despair. We have Social Security to help out and Medicare or Medicaid. In the Massachusetts township where I live, the publicly funded senior center provides so many engaging activities, both physical and intellectual, including even transportation, that no one over 50 need ever be lonely. I'm taking drumming and exercise classes there, playing chess, attending and sometimes moderating talks.

It provides community.

For we all need community. We need a group in which to belong.

One woman in my book group told us recently of a friend of hers, now in assisted living, who complained of her loneli-ness and the difficulty of finding true connections at this age.

"The tragedy is that no one knows me," she is reported to have said. "All they see is an old woman: all my experience sits unseen."

I have some sympathy, but it is tinged, I admit, with annoyance, wondering why she is not reaching out in curiosity to others, smiling and asking about themselves: Who are they? What are (or were) their interests, passions? What was the most astonishing or frightening or thrilling event in their lives? If she were to fill herself with the stories from others, could she possibly be lonely?

It has been pretty well proven that paying too much attention to social media, where you read the happy posts of strangers and friends, creates dissatisfaction and self-dislike. You cannot help but make comparisons, yet much of what we read on social media are half-truths and equivocations, or even downright lies, for who writes publicly about their terror and night sweats, their depression, or their hurt or unhappiness with their children or their lives? This recognition is why I fled Facebook in 2016—how unhappy it was making me, coupled with the concern that much of what I read in that presidential campaign year was utter fabrication. What can be trusted? I asked myself, when I didn't know who was behind the high-dudgeon pronouncements of Believe This! and Doubt That! When I couldn't tell who benefited from their beliefs? (Later it came out that much of these pronunciamentos were Russian robots, trolling to create election chaos.) I'm of the generation that learned to check the sources before crediting a truth.

All over the world people are lonely. And scared, and hungry and thirsty, and many without shelter. Millions struggle merely to stay alive in the face of drought, famine, floods, fires, violence, war, displacement, and diseases. They don't have time to be lonely. And for those like me, who live in the developed world and in a peaceful and liberal state of the union (which means a government that still works on behalf of its people), loneliness is a luxury. It was the poet Robert Bly who counseled at one poetry reading that if you feel lonely, you must go away alone, preferably to a cabin in the wilderness.

"Eat loneliness," he advised the audience before picking up his bouzouki to accompany another of his new poems.

Better yet, pick up the phone. Call a friend. "I'm feeling lonely," you say. "Come have coffee with me. We can do a banana-gram."

There is no shame in feeling loneliness. Just as there's no shame in anxiety. As long as we are alive, we will feel all the "negative" or discomfiting emotions as well as pleasant ones.

We call them "negative." But without judgment and resistance, they are merely signs indicating to us that some action might be good. Loneliness, anxiety, insecurity, a sense of inadequacy—they are merely part of being alive, as everyone feels separate sometimes, from nature and from our purpose and our community. And separate from God. From the mystery of who we are.

I once interviewed Sir Peter Scott, son of Robert Falcon Scott, the Antarctic explorer, who died when little Peter was only 2. Sir Peter was an enthusiastic ornithologist, conservationist, painter, athlete, yachter, Olympic and America's Cup sailor, and founder of the World Wildlife Fund for Nature. He was instrumental in shifting the policy of the International Whaling Commission to save endangered whales.

Imagine how surprised I was when he announced vehemently during our interview that "people are not flock animals. We're supposed to be alone."

It's one of my regrets that I didn't question this astonishing statement from a man who well knew how to be with and influence others. I was just a young girl at the time, awed by the Great Man, and I did not argue that actually we are herd animals: we need to belong, to be part of the pack, and we often feel best when we're in the middle, protected by the pack.

With my novelist ear, I make up stories of why he'd rather be alone.

I wonder whether men are lonelier than women. They have been taught to talk of indifferent topics like sports or politics. But put two women together and immediately they babble intimately of what's on their heart. I wonder about the boys who buy a machine gun to enter a school like commandos and spray little toddlers with bullets. I wonder how lonely they must have been.

A vast gulf separates loneliness and solitude. If you doubt me, try a crowded party where you hardly know anyone and the man you are talking to is casting his eyes like a fishing rod over your shoulder to find someone more important to dump you for.

Two possibilities exist: either we are
alone in the Universe or we are not.
Both are equally terrifying.

—Arthur C. Clarke, *Philosophy for the 21st Century*

For me, loneliness is a signal of being separate from my center and also separate from love—I've forgotten love, and that includes love for my poor, weak self as well as for others. Then I pray with an anxious, inadequate cry. (Beloved, help me, help!)

If we can't be with our pack, we need nature. Robert Bly was right about that. We need to walk in the woods, to finger the grooved bark of trees, to listen for ten or thirty minutes to the running water of a stream, or to sit for thirty minutes before a waterfall. Just being alone in nature changes our brain waves from the frenzy of perseverating beta waves to the slower, calming alpha waves and even to the deeper meditative brain waves that offer intuition, psychic experiences, telepathy, ESP, and more. It is when using the deeper brain waves that I am able intuitively to hear what a horse or cat is telling me. In my experience at this level, I am never lonely.

I remember in my childhood my gregarious father deliberately teaching my sister and me how to handle a party where we didn't know anybody, how (as they say) "to work a room." In those days people gave parties. I hardly go to parties anymore, but at 17 or 18 we "came out" with debutante parties to introduce us to society. It was actually a kind of marriage market to introduce us to appropriate young men whom at 18 or 20 we would marry and start a family with: the accepted role of women then. The Season began with a month of parties, tea dances, dinners, and late dances running from ten at night until two in the morning and ending with scrambled egg breakfasts for hungry, tired guests who might crawl home at four o'clock.

"Wait. Let me see you," my father said as we headed out dressed in cocktail dresses or full ball gowns. "You look lovely. Now remember. Don't just plunge into the room. Stand at the doorway, toss up your chin, and say to yourself, 'I am the most beautiful girl here,' and only then go in."

He gave other advice. "Compliment the boys. Boys are really scared. Find something nice to say, even if it's just 'I like your tie.'"

He said, "If you're shy, remember that everyone else is just as scared. Find someone in the room who looks lost and go to talk to them. Put them at ease. Make them feel better. Every guest has a duty to the hostess to help make her party fun."

Preach the Gospel at all times.
If necessary, use words.
—St. Francis of Assisi

It was good advice. Whenever I'm thinking of someone else, whenever I'm working for a cause, whenever I feel in service to something or someone besides myself, I am never lonesome. I think loneliness is a signal that I have disconnected from my Self. To connect, I have to be vulnerable, exposing myself to others and especially to myself, and here's the irony: only when I am openly vulnerable can people step forward to love and hold me. Only when I am vulnerable do I give them permission to open their hearts to me.

One last story, Eleanor. It's interesting that every enlightened or evolved person I have ever met or read about is overflowing with joy. They are laughing all the time. I remember meeting the Dalai Lama when I went to Dharamshala to interview him. He was saying goodbye to a man at the far end of an open colonnade at his working offices. He glanced around, saw me, and strode toward me in long steps, hands extended, with a beaming smile.

"Hello." He grabbed my hand and, holding tight, led me into his office. He settled me, still holding my hand, on the sofa and took a chair. "Now, how can I help you?" he asked, still patting my hand.

"Wow," I thought to myself. "That's the way I want to be greeted. Why was I taught such English reserve?" His joy spilled out over me in waves of energy.

I have never forgotten.

Oh No!

Dear Eleanor,

You know how much I've been looking forward to seeing you in only a few days when I could finally be in Paris again with you and the family.

It won't happen. A few days ago, I had such a pain in my calf that it forced me to take small steps and even to stop at times to shake out the cramp. After four days of waiting for things to work themselves out, I finally called the doctor. By then, being the weekend, I was sent to urgent care, which sent me urgently to the ER.

"You are to drive there right now," said the nurse. "Do not wait until tomorrow. You need another ultrasound. We are calling now to alert them you're coming."

Who knew it was serious?

At the ER they found that two blood clots in my leg have returned. I'm not allowed to step on a plane for at least six months, or more. They say if the clots move to the lungs, I could die from a pulmonary embolism or if to the brain, a stroke. I am back on blood thinner medications, this time for life, and, because of the blood thinners, if I scrape my knee or scratch a scab, blood pours like water, flowing down my leg or arm. Just banging my elbow raises a bruise; my forearms are purple with bruises.

This is my first real disorder. But look at the bright side: I don't have cancer or Parkinson's or Lou Gehrig's or MS. All I have are some deep-vein blood clots, which my body will absorb naturally in time while the blood thinner meds allow the blood to flow easily around the coagulated clots.

Still, I am dismayed. Is this the beginning of old-age troubles? They tell me I should not ride anymore. (As the doctor in the ER put it in horror: "YOU RIDE YOUR HORSE? Don't you know that if you hit your head while on blood thinners, you can start a brain bleed? We couldn't save you then.")

(For heaven's sake, I'm not going to hit my head. I use a helmet when I ride.)

Anyway, I shall not sit in the sun with you at our sidewalk café, chatting of this and that. It is one year since I started these letters to you. I wanted to talk about them and ask about how you feel now that you have walked through the gates of 60.

How old do you feel inside? I guess a youthful 35.

Please come to Massachusetts. I want to know your opinion of the Hollywood writers' strike.

Sophy

P.S. Since now I have time to write, I will add more to these letters. I want to tell about the Four Ages of our lives and what I have learned in the last 85 years.

Odd thoughts. Miscellaneous thoughts.

P.P.S. I can't finish without repeating a wonderful story told by my friend Margaret Dulaney in her book *Parables of Sunlight*. A man returned from a near-death experience to report what happened. He was met on the other side (he said) by a crowd of spirits, all of them talking excitedly.

"How was it?" they asked. "What happened?"

He had little to tell. He had failed at almost everything he tried, accomplished nothing important, but the more he told of his struggles, his failures, the more they crowded closer, exclaiming with delight:

"But you had a life! You had a Life!"

So yes, I've had a life. . . . I've been given my beautiful family and children, the perfect dog, one exquisite cat, my beloved horse. Such gifts . . . I keep on learning. I have only maybe ten more years to spend adoring this planet, this Eden, this school of suffering and compassion, this place on which to pour out love.

May you be happy and well, Eleanor. You're having a life!

Love, Gophy

PART 4

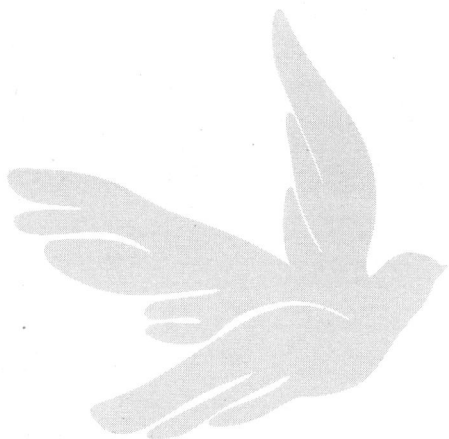

Four Ages of Life

Dearest Eleanor,

The gloomy philosopher Jaques in Shakespeare's *As You Like It* names desolately the seven ages of man: infant, schoolboy, lover, soldier, justice, drooling ancient, and helpless old age. But I find only four—four distinct ages (stages), each covering roughly 21 years. And now I'll tell you how I can defend my claim:

On the night before my 21st birthday, I sat at the little beat-up desk in my college dorm, staring out the window at the dark night, then picked up my pen and began a letter to myself, to be opened twenty-one years later at age 42. In it, I tried to set down in a few words who I was (filled with desires, self-examination), the meaning and purpose of life, my hopes for my future self, and my wish that she would have had a good and happy life. I really wanted the very best for that future woman. Who would be me.

When I was 42, before I opened that letter from my younger self, I wrote another, to be opened in twenty-one years at the age of 63. This second letter, written at age 42, was much longer than the first, for by then I was a successful writer and writing came easily, and also a lot had happened in those years that seemed as mysterious and magical, as if I lived in a fairy tale. I reported three transcendent experiences. Were there really angels, invisible forces intervening on my behalf? I had more questions at 42 than I could have imagined at 21, when in my arrogance I thought that I knew a lot. At 42, confused and conflicted, I was the mother of teenagers and moving toward divorce.

At 42, I felt I was walking blindfolded and barefoot down a gravel road, testing the path with my feet. At first, I often plunged into the sharp briars and thickets on the verge, only to overcompensate in my efforts to find the center of the road and lunge instead into the thorns on the opposite shoulder—until I learned to sense the silken reins of intuition, the guidance that I still feel comes from Elsewhere, something loving me. Today, no longer needing an electric cattle prod, I feel the slightest intuitive touch.

Looking back in hindsight, I could see the path illuminated, the story making sense; ahead the path was black as tar. The only thing to do was trust.

At 63, I wrote my third letter to myself, to be opened at age 84, and in this one I couldn't wait to tell my future self everything I'd learned in all these years. I had so much to say that this letter grew into three, at 63.

Finally, last year at age 84, I wrote my last letter to myself, and although I will likely not live to read it, I folded it neatly with the others in a small tin box on the book-shelf in my office. At 84, I found myself writing more to my young selves than to the woman I might become at 105. But all the letters, every one, are about being tender and kind toward ourselves and about daring to dive into the world.

Love letters to myself.

Curiously, what I had to say at 84 is not much different from what I wrote at 21. I remember that at 21 my modest injunction to myself was simply to do no harm. (To do good felt overly ambitious; even then I understood the gulf dividing intention and execution.) At 84, I did not wish myself a happy future or easy death. Instead, writing to the brave young women I had been and who had struggled at 21, 42, and 63 on their journeys, sometimes without even proper tools in their kit, I offered generosity and admiration, reminding them that all that is required of us is purity of intent. What happens to our bumbling efforts or how others receive them is not our responsibility. Only intention, only motive, matters. I urged my younger selves (which I guess is myself today) to forgive themselves for failing, for falling into fear, greed, pride, or for struggling awkwardly for status or safety or honors, or the desire to hide even from themselves the depths of our fear and inadequacy.

To forgive ourselves does not mean to forget, or to put ourselves back in an ugly or dangerous situation. It means to drop the rocks of regret and resentment and move on, emotionally liberated. Free. After forgiving our own failings, we may as well forgive everyone else as well, even the ones we fear or hate. (Often the same.)

Forgiveness is not an occasional act;
it is a permanent attitude.

—Martin Luther King Jr., Acceptance Speech,
Nobel Peace Prize, 1964

I find it annoying that Christ enjoined us to forgive but never talked about HOW. The Buddha, five hundred years earlier, gave precise instructions in the loving-kindness or Metta prayer, which is also found, I'm told, in ancient Hindu and Jain texts. It is said that the Buddha spent two hours a day slowly and with intention repeating the beautiful Metta. There are lots of variations. I know that you, Eleanor, a practicing Buddhist, already know this, but I can't help imposing, in the fashion of old folks, my favorite of many versions of the Metta prayer. (See below.) (Or don't.)

There is such suffering in the world that life seems more tragedy than comedy. The tragedy is that we love each other. We grieve at the loss of love. We are torn to shreds by life. We try to drown ourselves in alcohol or drugs or violence and war, to bend and numb our brains from the intensity of our feelings and fear. And all the while the Universe is loving, warming, comforting, healing, holding us, and all the while the beat of its dance of joy is rising, the drumbeat pounding in our ancient ears.

Only as I have gotten older have I seen the *lila*, heard the laughter.

After all these decades I have come to believe in the essential goodness in the Universe, that Something Out There—call it our angels, our guides—wants more and better for us than we can possibly imagine. The task is aways to let go, to surrender our self-reliance to IT (however we understand it). To trust, which is to say, choose Love.

It is a choice.

Basically all my wisdom, if there is any, comes from the brilliant men and women before me, for we are all dependent, interconnected, and I don't see that we've learned much in the last two or three thousand years. To love what you are doing and the people around you with all your mind and heart and being; and to act with fearless authenticity; and, if you can, to create, make art, or practice music—this is happiness, and it's a gift that doesn't have to come with age. But once past menopause and sensual, entrancing beauty, we become with all our scars and wrinkles both male and female, power and grace. We are still creative, though no longer bearing and rearing babies. Now we have time and energy to tackle cultural warts. We are greater than our younger selves, and if I were a poet, I would suggest that we become at this age like an ancient towering tree, silent with the depths and heights of knowledge we haven't even words to express.

Distilled from those sacramental fancies of my childhood has come the conviction that the nearest humanity approaches to perfection is in the persons of good women— and especially perhaps in the persons of kind, intelligent, and healthy women of a certain age, no longer shackled by the mechanisms of sex but creative still in other kinds, aware still in their love and sensuality, graceful in experience, past ambition but never beyond aspiration. In all countries among all races, on the whole these are the people I most admire: and it is into their ranks, I flatter myself, . . . that I have now admitted myself.
—Jan Morris, *Conundrum*

We all have stories, every one of us. We all are asked to tell our stories, to write them, speak them, whisper them to the indifferent walls. We are all pushed to answer the searing questions: Who am I? Why am I here? Only in our stories can the answers be found. Tell your stories, Eleanor. Tell them to your friends and sons and daughters. Tell them to yourself. Until you slowly learn the answers.

Meanwhile, it takes years to recognize the goodness, the kindness and creativity evident even in our wasteland of suffering and horror. But goodness lies all around us. It's found in tiny little daily moments, nothing special, yet each one unforgettable. Like the door held open for you unexpectedly, like the man who runs your suitcase up the subway stairs then continues, to his own inconvenience, carrying it to your train. Like the sunlight on a sidewalk café in Paris and the espresso in its doll-sized cup. Like the smile of blue braces and someone calling you honey, and the hope that they imply. Like an Egyptian princess disguised as a homeless person standing with you in the CVS.

Tiny moments of eternity and truth. In the face of such majesty, only silence prevails.

Just love yourself, Eleanor—not the narcissistic reflection of who you think other people think you should be but your whole self, good and bad, light and shadow, ideal and struggles.

Maybe that's the secret of a happy life. Just love.

What I Have Learned

Dearest Eleanor,

I've been thinking of what I've learned in more than eighty-five years of living, and of course there's too much even to set down, beginning, for instance, with learning after many decades to shut my mouth, zip my lips. So very much does not need to be said.

But upon reflection I have only three important things to pass on:

- All living things are sentient, with thoughts and consciousness
- The Dark Side
- We are beings of Light

All Living Things Are Sentient

Once in Belize, while touring an ancient Mayan ruin, my eye was captured by a spectacular tree on a nearby hill. So beautiful was this unusual tree that, leaving the group, I climbed the grassy hillside to approach the tree in admiration. Suddenly, as if a hand had hit my chest, I was forcibly stopped. I felt if I took one step closer, the tree would have murdered me (if it could), heaving a branch onto my head. You'll say it was my imagination. I thought so, too, but I stopped respectfully, a little frightened by the open anger of the tree. Listening, I sent a heart-thought outward, asking permission to approach.

It refused. I have known trees to be welcoming or most commonly indifferent, but this is the only tree I have ever met that raged with pain and hate. Bowing, I returned to my group.

"What kind of tree is that?" I asked the guide, pointing up the hill. "I've never seen one like that. It's magnificent."

"It's a mahogany," he told me. "Very valuable. Once this whole area was mahogany forest." He shrugged. "It was completely logged. Long ago. That's the only one left. It must have been a sapling when the other trees were cut and hauled away."

Surely, when we walk in the woods, we come away restored by the spiritual energy of the towering, silent trees. Scientists have now discovered that trees communicate with each other in their own alien language. Trees count; they remember; they nurse sick neighbors, signal danger to other trees, feed and tend their young, including the sprouts of other

species. I'm told they keep the stumps of felled companions alive for centuries by feeding them a sugar solution
through their own root system. I cannot help but believe
trees scream when cut. And that nearby trees shrink back in
anguish and in fear.

I'm sure they love.

All living things are sentient. Beetles and flies and the
tiny ants in my kitchen that pause even when rushing to
touch antennae, greeting each other, passing along their
queen scent (are you in my tribe?) as they churn on their
indefatigable path—even the smallest ants feel fear and love
and relief. The patient spider spinning her exquisite web has
emotions, probably just like mine. We send rockets to look
for life on Mars, yet all the while we ignore that all around
us the earth itself and all its creatures are singing in tones
we cannot hear of loneliness and fear, longing and loss,
beauty and love.

Of course, they also understand death. I'm always
amazed when scientists discover that animals have a sense
of humor, or love one another, or talk to one another, or call
each other by name. They are sentient! When her beloved
dog died, my daughter brought her cat into the room to see
the body of his friend. The cat pitta-patted to the dead dog,

sniffed it, then lay, curling into the embrace of the cooling corpse, his head against its neck, body on body. The cat lay there for a few moments, then rose, shook itself, and stalked away. He had said goodbye.

I remember years ago how my tame rabbit wept when her kits were killed. And we think that animals have no sense of death! Of grief. Or love. Or loss.

Oh, humans!

We can be so ignorant.

The Dark Side

Once I was reading in bed, lost in the story, when suddenly PLOP, a weight landed on my chest. I was flattened. Paralyzed. I could not move. It was black as tar. It had long claws or talons and a grimacing, sharp-toothed smile as it peered about. It was a well of loneliness and filled with fear, rage, hostility.

I lay horrified, helpless. It was only an imp, but it was so powerfully the expression of pure loneliness, darkness, and fear that it filled and terrified me. I say I could not move, but with the tip of my index finger I made an infinitesimal sign of the cross.

WOOSH! It was gone.

What had happened? I rose from the bed and walked around my room uneasily. I felt dirty, frightened, out of sorts.

I went in the bathroom to wash myself, shaken, weepy, and I realized I had just seen the epitome of evil, and it was named Fear. It was loneliness beyond belief. It was the utter and devastating absence of love.

It was horrible, a Thing, and I wondered whether we should be praying for the imps and demons, too, poor things, experiencing an eternity of that. I think we should probably all be praying for them, sending them into the Light.

Of course there is a Dark Side, Eleanor. I have seen it more than once. It lies grinning all around us. I tell you only this:

- Don't dabble.
- Don't play with it. Never think you are big enough to take it on.
- In the face of the Dark Side, remember to place yourself instantly in God, by which I mean Love: "I belong to God" is enough to say, "I Love!" With that thought alone, the Dark Side will vanish.

We Are Beings of Light

The first time I saw people as light, surrounded by light and emitting light, I was in the San José airport in Costa Rica, and it so affected me that I had to put on sunglasses to hide the tears seeping down my cheeks. Here was a moving, milling, noisy crowd of tourists, passengers, porters pushing suitcases, women with babies, native women in bright costumes, soldiers carrying rifles, pilots, staff, and flight attendants—and the noise: don't forget the rumble of voices, loudspeaker announcements, and feet—a waterfall of sound.

Suddenly, a great silence fell over me, and in that silence, I saw that each person sitting, walking, standing, moving—everyone—was shining with light. Enveloped by light. Haloed with light.

"This is how God sees us," I thought, and I sat in that well of silence overcome by the beauty of us humans.

Later, on Machu Picchu, I was offered a shattering mystical revelation (Moses on the mountaintop) when, coming slowly out of it, I saw light, like lasers, pouring off the palms of my hands—and not only off my hands and skin but off of everything. Every living thing was streaming with light: the grasses, the trees, the injured dog limping past, the bus driver, my fellow tourists all chatting over their pisco sours, oblivious to their light or the light of others, oblivious to how their energy fields shook out waves in the light of others passing by. All living things are beings of light, haloed, as we walk about oblivious.

It is the light of love.

These days I can see it when I try. Anyone can. Don't gaze at the form or face. With soft-focused eyes, look at the empty space around the person's head. Look at the triangle of space at someone's head and shoulders. Or look a foot or more above the person's head. Can you catch a shimmering, like heat waves rising on hot tar in summer? It is easiest to see in soft light or semi-dusk and against a plain background or blank wall. Don't try to find it in sunlight or against a splash of splotchy colors. If you don't see it, lift your gaze higher. Some people's auras extend ten feet above and around them.

Of course you'll think it's your imagination. You'll think you need to have your eyes checked. Look again. Look often.

Many of us sense this spiritual energy. "I'm beside myself," we murmur. And indeed we are. The light of our energy field has shifted awkwardly askew, hanging off to one side. We feel "out of sorts," uncentered. Take a deep breath, expel it through your mouth, then consciously bring your energy back to center.

When you are loving, your light expands, enormous. The bride walking down the aisle is shining. "She's in love," we say, instinctively recognizing the light.

When someone is angry, his energy shoots out in sharp daggers and flying knives, and anyone empathic will feel it, like being whipped with barbed wire, even when the anger is not directed at them.

When frightened or depressed, the light shrinks inward protectively, as if the energy has wilted or is dragging heavily behind. (This is also true for people on drugs: their auras go amiss, contorted, dim.)

Animals have auras, too—all living things.

Even the trees have auras. Look at the spaces between the branches. Even your enemy, or someone whom you find particularly annoying, is a being of light, doing the best they can in a difficult world.

Looking shifts my perspective, for this aura can be seen only by putting aside momentarily our other gifts, our analytical, critical faculties of judgment and discernment.

For a few moments you see with spiritual eyes, unguarded.

Letters to Myself

Dear Eleanor,

When rereading these letters, I was especially struck by the one I wrote at 21 on fine letter paper, written front and back by hand in black ink and sent in a matching envelope inscribed to: "Miss Penny Doub, to be opened on her 42nd birthday 21 years from now." (Penny was my affectionate nickname in those days, before my husband, David, managed to take back my given name and change the surname, too.) I am impressed by the formality of the letter and the fact that not a word was scratched out or changed. Looking at the deeply slanted black writing, with its vaulting highs and lows, the slender calligraphy, I felt I had touched a different century. And of course I have, for I'm reading them in 2024.

The second letter, written at 42, is many pages long, typed this time, and again with nothing crossed out or changed. The third, at 63, written in 1999, is actually four letters, all written by hand in ink, at different times. At 63, I couldn't stop writing. So I give you excerpts from these. The last, at 84, was written on the computer.

But none has the formality of that precious first. I am intrigued that none of the later ones speak of my husband of twenty years or my beloved children or my parents or sister in France, or friends, or my work—all the things I love and that you'd think I'd write about.

Be kind. These were never written for publication. I have edited lightly, cutting for repetition or discretion, but no significant changes have been made.

Sophy Burnham
(aka Penny)

Letter to Myself at 21, to Be Opened at 42

12.12.1957

Tomorrow is my 21st birthday, and I write this letter now, not because I feel any burning need to record my thoughts in the last hour of my twentieth age, but rather because someday I might be interested in them: I know how I wish I had done it when I was in Europe.

What do I feel now? What am I? I don't know.

First, I want to note that I hate self-analysis and I loathe the petty disrupture of a whole palpably living thing into tiny pieces; yet I find that I am continually analyzing myself, every thought, every action, every grimace . . . Self-analysis can be dangerous: it is certainly a sign of egoism; it proves nothing. But, as of now, I have been a slave to it.

I find that I am no lover of truth. I don't care if a thing be true or false; I love being right, hate being wrong. And this only because I love admiration.

Everything I do is aimed in some way, it seems, to gain me admiration. I write a thesis not because I long for higher learning, nor specialized studies, nor cum laude, but simply for its prestige! That is why I like to charm people: admiration. Unfortunately, since my desire does not extend to all people, I often can't be bothered to make the effort to charm . . .

No matter how well you do a thing (and this I must remember!), no matter how good you are, there is always someone better. You can speak a foreign language and understand two others, but there are some who speak ten languages fluently . . . I must not want too much and must not be depressed with myself.

Right now I am torn by desires: I suppose that I have always been, and always will be—I can't really remember. But now I want more things than I have ever desired in my life. So it seems. I still want to live someplace where I can be surrounded by all my friends and know that they will stay. Death I do not think of yet. I'm afraid a fear of death will come to me as I grow older—

I want to travel . . . all over the world, and inquire into things and investigate for myself, see new places and strange customs: the East . . . I want to return to Italy . . . I want to live one winter in New York, going to parties, and work there of course, because otherwise I might be bored—I'd like to spend one entire winter as a ski bum . . . I want to get married.

Why? Why marry? To take care of someone whom I love and who loves me. That's all. That's enough . . .

It is now past midnight. I can say I am 21 . . . I feel calm, perhaps too calm and too sure of myself. Alas! A sign of maturing. La Signora [whom I lived with in Italy] would hardly recognize me, I don't think, from the flighty, fun-loving, laughing, often thoughtless me of last year . . .

The most important thing in the world is to do no harm (if you can). And think of others. Any time you are depressed or furious or defeated, look around you at two things: the world—a sparrow, a twig, the sky, ice, a leaf—and the people around you. If your depression continues, find some way to do something for someone else.

I hope your life is as nice from now on as it has been up to now; may it hold even more adventures and may happiness be yours. Give love.

Penny

Letter to Myself, Written at 42, to Be Opened at 63

Dear Gophy,

I write this on a beautiful warm brilliant blue fall day. In two months I will be 42. Years ago, at 21, I wrote myself a letter, to be opened 21 years later. I don't remember what is in that. But I begin this letter now, to be sealed and put away before opening that Voice from the past . . .

Will I have changed? I'm now married with children. I'm still filled with longings.

I want to set down here three things that have happened in my life, three things that changed me. The first is how an angel saved my life; the second is a dream that I once had in which I died; the third is what happened when I was blinded by God . . .

Now, about the meaning of life: I don't know much.

Once I thought what I wanted from life was to Understand. And I mean everything. All of life. Each person, each bug and beast: just understand.

There have been moments when I felt I did—with a wondering gasp of comprehension—so that was it! . . .

And sometimes I have felt that I held the meaning of life just there in the cup of my hands. All I needed was to reach out with enough openness of heart, with enough intellectual analysis, acuity, discipline, yearning—and I would touch the Center of It All. It would be (in capitals) Unity. To understand totally is to be so absorbed with Unity that object and subject become one and the same. To understand is to dip into the absence of separateness, the very quality that demands the longing to understand.

Of course I have experienced this terrible separateness. It is perhaps the howling lonely haunting fear at the core of all humans, the realization that ultimately we are alone. It is the aloneness that makes us hide behind empty form, that creates stop-think patterns of behavior, repression, the shells of social masks that, if stripped away, leave us naked and so vulnerable that the only relief lies in going mad.

But I have also experienced the absence of separation—a flash, a single instant: satori, nirvana. I have seen the face of God and worshipped at the one-ness of the Universe. I have lived as long as two weeks exalted by divine light. I have seen pure light streaming through the air and heard the singing of the planets in ethereal realms. ("Look! Look at the light!" But no one else could see.) It happened in the spring of 1976 after surgery in Massachusetts General Hospital, and it continued for more than a week after my return home, two weeks in all. Then slowly it passed away like water running through a sieve, because no one can remain in that exalted state for long, going mad in praise of God, leaving everything for God: without food or drink or work or duty, but merely living in Divine Light. I thought, "I would give my soul to hold onto that light," and then realized I'd been given it. The joke is (ha ha!) we do not need to lose our soul to see that, but to find it. There you have it. That is the whole of it, and I am certain that when we die, we are there again, one with the Light, the Divine. Having experienced it, I cannot look at death as anything but a joyous occasion, the rebirth indeed after the death-in-life of this life-form.

That vision changed my life. When my mother died this summer, my first reaction was of joy, that she should experience this Light. It was only later that I wept with the terror of my own aloneness, for that is part of living: sorrow at the parting, the loss of my friend and antagonist. This matter of my mother, however, is complex. I wept also at being clawed to undertake her work, which is not mine, to keep up the family property, to care for Daddy [stroke], duties that infringe on my own responsibilities to my own family and my life. I am still coping with that and wait to see the outcome.

What is the purpose of life?

There was a time when I would have answered glibly and with youthful enthusiasm that the answer was to serve others.

I do not live by that rule now, although I give it lip service. I live for myself in the most selfish form imaginable . . .

There are things I want . . . I want to write (which is my one talent) and dear God, let me be strong enough, perceptive enough to see . . . Give me the talent to find words that reach out, touch another. Give me the courage to try, and when I fail, to try again.

I write this at a table at CCNY one afternoon between appointments. As I typed those words, the man at the next table stood up, supported by his crutch, looked at me, and said, "Ah, that first step is the hardest one."

What I'm trying to say is this "I" is no more than you. I am thee; you are me. We live isolated by our forms, our sex, our social class, our knowledge and the degrees of talent, intellect, articulation in our systems. In isolation we reach out to each other with one great cry, all of humanity singing: I love you. And sometimes it shouts: I can't hear you. Tell me you love me. I'm frightened. Do you love me?

This is the Janus-face of humankind, balanced between yes and no, fear-hope, optimism-pessimism, fullness-emptiness, openness-closedness. Love: I think that is the most magnanimous word of all, the first word, pronounced at the very beginning of the Bang.

LOVE,
Gophy

Letter to Myself, Written at 63, to Be Opened at 84

12/09/99

My dearest Penny,

Sophy—

This is probably the last letter you will read from me, who is yourself of twenty-one years ago; and I wish I could be writing to you on 12.12.99—your birthday, my birthday. But this year I will be in New York on Saturday night, and I don't trust that I will be free to write to you.

. . . I love you. Are you happy? Are you still healthy and optimistic, and do you laugh freely and explore and try new things? Are you good-hearted? And do you still love people and do they find themselves attracted to you? Do you still write? Or have you retired now? I want to know all about you, though in truth I can wait to learn . . . Tonight I sit at my desk, here at 1405 31st Street, and I can think of nothing important to tell you about myself. Or life. Considering this lovely world, I understand less now at 63 than I understood almost a quarter century ago.

For some reason the image of a hand lifted in blessing, open palmed and blessing you.

. . . Beyond that I leave the blankness of the [rest of the] page. All love.

Only love,
Gophy

A second letter written later:

Dear Gophy-to-be—

Greetings. How are you? I hope you are well and healthy, and particularly I hope you are happy—happy with a deep runnel of joy . . . The cat is curled behind me on my chair, and I write now on the computer since my handwriting is nearly illegible these days.

I wonder if you found the partner of your dreams. I hope so, for it means that I will find it, too! I wish you beautiful memories, much love in your life—wisdom—enlightenment. I wish you have a radiant, luminous presence—and I wish that your life has touched those around you in wild wonderful mysterious and joyful ways.

Until this evening I was wrapped in a depression. It started a week (or a month) ago and yesterday was so serious that I began and ended the day in tears. Last night, determined to stop, I took St. John's wort and exercised (one and a half-hour's dance class). I am careful to see people and to sit under my light-box . . .

Yesterday I knelt in the bathtub under the pouring shower and prayed to be relieved . . . and a few hours later voilà! The depression lifted.

Tomorrow I am 63. The depression fell at being old. Adumbrated. Used up. The government tells me I am old—while inside I still feel, young, sexy, desirable. I am afraid, because what if it's true, that people are not loved or desirable or useful after a certain age? That is why I send you, at 84, all, and I mean ALL, deep love.

Sophy Burnham—Penny

Letter to Myself at 84,
to Be Opened at 109

December 12, 2020

Surely, this is the last of the four letters I shall write myself every twenty-one years. I think I am writing this time not to my future self but to my own self, long past. As I look toward my birthday next week, I remember my grandmother musing on her 80th at the birthday party with the family gathered at the farm. "It's all gone so fast," she murmured. As a young girl I snickered, having no idea what she meant, because my own life was moving slowly still, with each exciting moment engraved in my mind and heart. Now I know what she meant. It's gone so fast. And there has been so much in it.

What a life! What a world! It has been so rich, so abundant, bountiful, inexorable, inevitable, so filled with grace.

Had I imagined at the age of 20 or 21 what I'd have liked to have happen, my wildest dreams, I would have done myself a disservice. I could not have conceived of the miraculous joys and delights that have been spread before me: a banquet of tastes and sounds, of sorrow and grief, hope, comfort, encouragement, experiences, and love, and love poured upon me by grace alone . . . I am weeping as I write this, my heart overflowing with humility and gratitude . . .

From my high footing at this age, looking out over wider horizons, I find myself filled with regrets and remorse for things I've said and done, or for ones I've not said or done when I should have; and this is coupled with a curious compassion for the ignorant, unskillful girl who thought she was doing it all so well. (Not that I'm so skillful now, but you can't help but learn a few things over the years.) Maybe it's to that young self I'm writing, or maybe to myself now.

Here's the thing: I don't know anything.

Docie, my beloved mother-in-law, told me. "I used to think I knew so much," she murmured, "and now I don't know anything."

That's the way I feel. How can I have so much to learn after all these years?

Nonetheless, there are a few things I've learned in all these years. And as an aside, I add that I love this life. I'm not ready to die yet. I want another whole lifetime to adore the beauty of nature, the goodness of people, who are all struggling as best they can with traumas and difficulties, with stress, fear, ignorance (the lack of tools in the toolbox they were given), but with a sweetness of soul which flashes helplessly out as violence and hate. We are inherently good. All of us.

We all need forgiveness. So hard. Sometimes all we can do is pray for the willingness to forgive, and our prayers at first may be short and simple ("Dear God, give the bastard what he deserves!"). As you continue trying, though, praying and wanting to forgive the one who has offended you, wanting the best for this person who has radically hurt you, you find yourself gradually healing, and you find the hurt is slowly diminishing.

To forgive does not mean you forget or put yourself back into the same unhealthy situations. Neither does it mean that you approve of the offense. It means that you choose to live without hatred and fear dragging at your life. You choose the path to happiness. You condemn injustice, and still you can have compassion for the tortured creature who perpetuated it. I think it was Pascal who wrote that to understand is to forgive.

So my questions to myself are: How can I be more awake? How can I be more present to this miracle of my life?

Two days later: Today I am down, blue, paralyzed by inertia. I've known it before. All my life I have had these sharp and sudden collapses of energy in which, as if a veil has been tossed over me, I see darkly, without rejoicing or clarity or thanks. When I was young, these moods lasted for days, and now, thankfully, only hours. Yet still, they descend over me, this sudden collapse of energy. Last night I slept poorly, waking every hour with cramps in my legs and toes. Today I am fighting an inner conflict. My 84th birthday is coming up on Saturday, and I am in combat with my age. I feel inside about age 50—and then I'm confronted by the reality of years. I'm old. I look at friends my age, and I'm brought up short by wrinkles and rhytidomes of age: I'm horrified. "That's how I look," I think. Inside I am youthful, sensual, still desirable, springing forward with joy and delight. But everything in my culture says I am finished, ugly, worthless, old. What I want is to be loved and even desired by a man, but how could anyone want me when I look like that? When I look in the mirror, I see a face that's flat, without expression, without energy or light. What do others see? Alain calls from France or L. from Virginia (when he's drunk), telling me he wants to hold me in his arms, dance, kiss. I dismiss them both. They're in their cups.

All my life I have been attractive to men. I'm accustomed to being admired. I'm vain. And yes. I want to be sensually desired instead of being a withered wisdom-woman, a hunchbacked crone. Mind you, I have hated my age all my life long. I was ashamed at 25, at 30, at 44. And that is due to cultural conditioning, because everything we read or see tells us we're not good enough, young enough, old enough, wise enough, strong enough, with beautiful enough skin or hair or muscle suppleness. Oh, this matter of aging! It's a bitch!

Of course I know the answer: Dive more deeply into this moment. Be present NOW. Don't let my thoughts affect my mood. Forgive. Forgive myself for living long or not well enough, or being less than the advertising beauty products shout that I could be if only I bought their creams, face lifts, Botox, facials . . . Another way of saying this: Accept it. Accept the years. Give up childish dreams of beauty being related somehow to happiness.

What I want to tell you, my darling, my little girl who once was me: will you listen?

You don't have to be perfect. We are all just humans. Where did we learn we're not enough? Where did we learn we had to be perfect? Or else that we had to accomplish something (a book, an invention or discovery, purchase of a house or land) in order to be loved? Where did I learn that being loved is more important than being filled with love ourselves, pouring it out in drenching waterfalls onto . . . everything.

. . . Just be happy. Worrying is a form of praying for what you want to have happen. Our thoughts are prayers. Watch your thoughts, my darling, and observe: are you asking or are you giving?

The only true prayer is for happiness.

Don't cast your fishing line into the pond of a future that has not happened yet. Don't make yourself miserable with imaginary fears or too many regrets at past mistakes. Mistakes are only messages about how to do it better next time.

Laugh every day.

Today Diane, Molly's friend in India, told her, "I hate the saying rest in peace. When you die, don't go peacefully into eternal rest. Forget resting in peace. Choose a life full of problems to solve and difficulties instead."

When Molly told me, I laughed out loud. All my dark thoughts (it had been a rough day) vanished. Yes, just live your life fearlessly, abundantly, good and bad.

I've been given such gifts . . . I have only maybe ten more years to spend adoring this planet, this Eden, this school of suffering and joy, this place on which to pour out love.

May you be happy and well, my future self. You've had a life.

Love,
Sophy

AFTER-WORDS

How to Forgive

Dear Eleanor,

I know that you, my dearest, already know the Metta prayer, but this is my favorite of its many forms.

May you be well and happy, free of suffering and pain. Liberated.

Sophy

Metta (in Pali), or "loving-kindness," describes a strong, sincere wish for the happiness of all beings. It is like the love of a mother who would give her life for her children. It includes the mother's own health, too, without which her children will not survive. I am told that the Buddha spent two hours a day slowly repeating this prayer. Take your time. It should take about twenty minutes to do the entire thing. If you have less time, then forgive YOURSELF, and during the day consider the rest of the prayer of loving-kindness when you can.

*Sit quietly. Calm your mind by taking a few slow
breaths—or more: perhaps you have already been
meditating for an hour before you begin. The outgoing
breath is twice as long as the intake. This loving-
kindness always begins with yourself. Speak the three
phrases silently to yourself, pondering them carefully.
At the pauses marked with three periods, wait, breathe,
considering, if possible, from the heart. Take a breath,
and Begin with Yourself:*

May I be forgiven for all offenses I have committed . . .
knowingly and unknowingly . . . by thought, word, and deed . . .
May I be forgiven of them all.
May I forgive all those who have offended me . . . knowingly
and unknowingly . . . by thought, word, and deed . . .
May I forgive them all . . .
May I be well and happy, free of suffering and pain . . .
Liberated.

*Now turn your attention to someone you love dearly—
a child or close friend, someone whom you love
unconditionally.*

May she be forgiven for all offenses she has committed . . .
knowingly and unknowingly by thought, word, and deed . . .

May she be forgiven of them all . . .
May she forgive all those who have offended her . . .
knowingly and unknowingly by thought, word, and deed . . .
May she forgive them all . . .
May she be well and happy, free of suffering and pain . . .
Liberated.

Now turn your attention to a stranger—the bus driver on
this morning's bus, the checkout clerk at the market, the
homeless beggar.

May this stranger be forgiven for all offenses he has
committed . . . knowingly and unknowingly . . . by thought,
word, and deed . . . May he be forgiven of them all . . .
May he forgive all those whom he has offended . . .
knowingly and unknowingly . . . by thought, word, and
deed . . . May he forgive them all . . .
May he be well and happy, free of suffering and pain . . .
Liberated.

Extend your energy field outward to a friend and repeat
the prayer, loving her.

Extend your energy field outward now to an enemy
or to someone whom you resent. If this is too difficult,

skip this step. Later, you will be able to include even your
so-called enemy.

May this person be forgiven for all offenses he has
committed . . . knowingly and unknowingly . . . by thought,
word, and deed . . . May he be forgiven of them all.
May this person forgive all those who have offended him . . .
knowingly and unknowingly . . . by thought, word, and deed.
May he forgive them all.
May he be well and happy . . . free of suffering and pain . . .
Liberated.

Now extend your heart energy outward to all sentient beings
in this city block or area.

May all beings in this area (or city or city block) be
forgiven, etc.
To all beings in this province or state: May all beings
in this state be forgiven . . . etc.

Now extend your heart even further, to all beings in this nation.

May all sentient beings in this country be forgiven . . . etc.

Now extend outward to include all beings in this hemisphere.

May all sentient beings in this hemisphere be
forgiven, etc.

*Now wrap your loving kindness around the globe, our
pretty planet, and send out your prayer.*

May all sentient beings on this pretty planet be forgiven
for all offenses, known etc. . . .
May they forgive all those who have offended them . . .
knowingly and unknowingly . . . etc.
May they be well and happy, free from suffering and pain.
May they be liberated.

*And finally, extend your energy out to the farthest stars,
to all spiritual beings known and unknown, visible and
invisible.*

May all sentient beings, known and unknown, visible
and invisible, be forgiven . . . of all offenses they have
committed knowingly and unknowingly . . . by thought,
word, and deed. May they be forgiven of them all.
May all sentient beings, visible and invisible, forgive . . .
all those who have offended them . . . knowingly and
unknowingly . . . by thought, word, and deed. May they
forgive them all.

May they be well and happy, free of suffering and pain, liberated.

Now sit. Feel your energy. Feel Love.

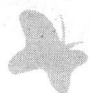

Acknowledgments

This is a work of nonfiction. Everything really happened and is true, insofar as the distortion of memory allows. Many of the people I would like to thank are dead, and if I were to name everyone who belonged in these acknowledgments, it would take a book of its own. But at the head of the list, high on the platform, stands Eleanor Coleman, my cousin, a film producer in Paris (and if you want to see her work and stand like me and Cortez, "silent on the peak in Darien," check out *Navozand, The Musician* on Paramount and now on Netflix). Without her question, this book would not have been born.

Next, my horse Spring, because her love keeps me sane when the world becomes too much, reminding me to stay right here, right now. She reminds me to slow down. Take a breath. Nothing can be accomplished in frenzy.

Moving to the more common acknowledgments, I thank my precious women's coven of white witches, Joyce Rosenfield, Margaret Humbolt-Droz, and Gayle Hudson, who even in advancing years stride on, affirming that artists create all our lives long. It is Joyce who insists on the first-person

singular instead of my shy avoidance with the generic "you."
Let's add also my writer's group with Gloria Squitiro, Candida
Deluise, and Lisa Thompson, who have been meeting with me
for ten or twelve years.

My dearest friends, Marie-Monique and Ray Steckel,
Judith Tartt, and Sarah Banker, friends for decades, have
consistently supported me, hands at my back whenever I grew
discouraged. And how can I forget in this list the support of
my sister, Anne Marzin, in Paris, the only person left alive
who shares my memories, or of my two daughters, Sarah
and Molly (the latter also a writer—of award-winning children's books, I shout proudly), both of whom bring me to
tears of love?

Many of my readers know that I believe in angels. I think
they were working on this publication, too. One day with the
first drafts finished, my friend the author Julia Cameron telephoned out of the blue from Santa Fe, to announce that her
agent would be good with me. How did she know I needed
a new literary agent? That mine, after thirty years, had
resigned? She introduced me to Susan Raihofer, and who
would not be captivated by this enthusiastic, intelligent, joyful
young woman? Without her delight, this book would never
have seen the light of day. Susan put me in contact with Patty
Rice, my editor, and it is Patty whose thoughtful editing and
kindness has touched my heart. No publisher of any of my

earlier books has ever asked my opinion about a cover or been so open in our relationship. I should like to add the copyeditor and the cover designer, except I don't know their names. So many people whose names I don't know. To each one,

Thank you.

Also by Sophy Burnham

NONFICTION

*The Art Crowd: The True Story of How
a Few Rich and/or Powerful Insiders
Control the World's Art Market*

*The Landed Gentry: Passions & Personalities
Inside America's Propertied Class*

*A Book of Angels: Reflections on Angels Past
and Present And True Stories of How They
Touch Our Lives*

Angel Letters

*The Ecstatic Journey: Walking the Mystical Path
in Everyday Life*

The Path of Prayer

The Art of Intuition: Cultivating Your Inner Wisdom

*For Writers Only: Inspiring Thoughts on the
Exquisite Pain and Heady Joy of the Writing
Life, from Its Greatest Practitioners*

NOVELS

Revelations

The Treasure of Montségur, a Story of the Cathars

The President's Angel

Love, Alba

YOUNG ADULT NOVELS
Buccaneer
The Dogwalker

POETRY
Falling: Love Struck, The God Poems

FILMS (FOR THE SMITHSONIAN INSTITUTION)
The Smithsonian's Whale
The Leaf Thieves
The Music of Shakespeare's England

PLAYS
*Penelope: The Story of the Odyssey from
Penelope's point of view*
Prometheus Bound by Aeschylus, translation
& adaptation by Sophy Burnham
Prometheus Released, by Sophy Burnham
The Study (aka, Snowstorms)
The Meaning of Life

CHILDREN'S RADIO PLAYS (NPR)
The Witch's Tale
Beauty and the Beast
The Nightingale